Healthy Recipes
Top 60 Soup and Salad Recipes

Learn How to Mix Different Ingredients to Create Tasty Meals and Build A
Complete Meal Plan For Your Diet

Jane Sommers

Table of Contents

1. Cabbage Diet Soup

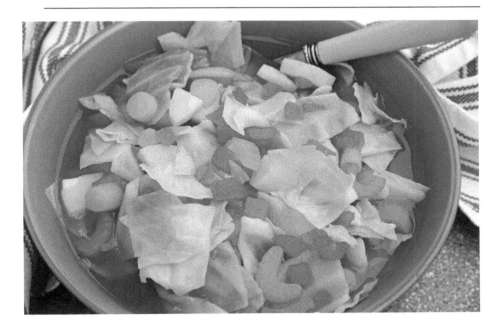

Active: 35 mins

Total: 55 mins

Servings: 6

Ingredients

- 2 tablespoons extra-virgin olive oil
- 1 medium onion, chopped
- 2 medium carrots, chopped
- 2 stalks celery, chopped
- 1 medium red bell pepper, chopped
- 2 cloves garlic, minced
- 1 ½ teaspoon Italian seasoning
- ½ teaspoon ground pepper
- ¼ teaspoon salt
- 8 cups low-sodium vegetable broth

5

- 1 medium head green cabbage, halved and sliced
- 1 large tomato, chopped
- 2 teaspoons white-wine vinegar

Instructions

- Heat oil in a large pot over medium heat. Add onion, carrots, and celery. Cook, stirring until the vegetables begin to soften, 6 to 8 minutes. Add bell pepper, garlic, Italian seasoning, pepper, and salt and cook, stirring, for 2 minutes.
- Add broth, cabbage, and tomato; increase the heat to medium-high and bring to a boil. Reduce heat to maintain a simmer, partially cover, and cook until all the vegetables are tender, 15 to 20 minutes more. Remove from heat and stir in vinegar.

Nutrition

- Calories: 133; Protein 3g; Carbohydrates 19.8g; Dietary Fiber 7g; Sugars 11g; Fat 5.2g; Saturated Fat 0.7g; Vitamin A Iu 4480.2IU; Vitamin C 88.2mg; Folate 91mcg; Calcium 110.7mg; Iron 1.5mg; Magnesium 30.2mg; Potassium 504.1mg; Sodium 451.1mg; Thiamin 0.1mg.

2.   Vegetable Weight-Loss Soup

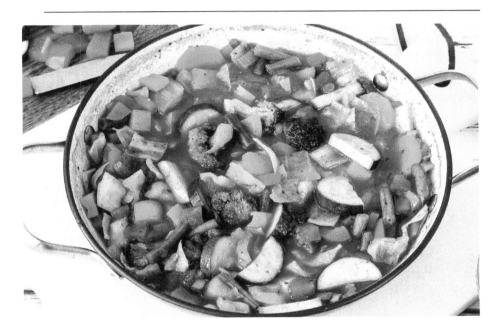

Active: 45 mins

Total: 1 hr

Servings: 8

Ingredient

- 2 tablespoons extra-virgin olive oil
- 1 medium onion, chopped
- 2 medium carrots, chopped
- 2 stalks celery, chopped
- 12 ounces fresh green beans, cut into 1/2-inch pieces
- 2 cloves garlic, minced
- 8 cups no-salt-added chicken broth or low-sodium vegetable broth

- 2 (15 ounces) cans of low-sodium cannellini or other white beans, rinsed
- 4 cups chopped kale
- 2 medium zucchini, chopped
- 4 Roma tomatoes, seeded and chopped
- 2 teaspoons red-wine vinegar
- ¾ teaspoon salt
- ½ teaspoon ground pepper
- 8 teaspoons prepared pesto

Instructions

- Heat oil in a large pot over medium-high heat. Add onion, carrot, celery, green beans, and garlic. Cook, stirring frequently until the vegetables begin to soften, about 10 minutes. Add broth and bring to a boil. Reduce heat to a simmer and cook, stirring occasionally, until the vegetables are soft, about 10 minutes more.
- Add white beans, kale, zucchini, tomatoes, vinegar, salt, and pepper. Increase heat to return to a simmer; cook until the zucchini and kale have softened, about 10 minutes. Top each serving of soup with 1 teaspoon pesto.

Nutrition

Calories: 225; Protein 12.7g; Carbohydrates 27.8g; Dietary Fiber 7.6g; Sugars 5.3g; Fat 8.4g; Saturated Fat 1.4g; Vitamin A Iu 4134.1IU; Vitamin C 30.3mg; Folate 52.3mcg; Calcium 106.4mg; Iron 3.1mg; Magnesium 88.6mg; Potassium 865.8mg; Sodium 406mg; Thiamin 0.7mg.

3. Italian Wedding Soup

Total: 1 hr 30 mins

Servings: 8

Ingredients

- Meatballs
- 1 pound ground turkey breast
- 1 cup fresh whole-wheat breadcrumbs
- 1 large egg, lightly beaten
- ¼ cup finely chopped fresh parsley
- 2 cloves garlic, minced
- 1 tablespoon Worcestershire sauce
- ½ teaspoon crushed fennel seeds
- ½ teaspoon freshly ground pepper
- ¼ teaspoon salt
- 2 teaspoons extra-virgin olive oil
- ½ cup dry white wine

Soup

- 1 tablespoon extra-virgin olive oil
- 1 cup chopped onion (1 medium)
- 1 cup chopped carrots (2 medium)
- 1 cup chopped celery (2 medium stalks)
- 4 cups chopped cabbage (about 1/2 small head)
- 8 cups low-sodium chicken broth
- 1 15-ounce can white beans, rinsed
- 8 cups coarsely chopped escarole or thinly sliced kale leaves (about 1 bunch)
- ½ cup freshly grated Romano cheese

Instructions

- To prepare meatballs: Combine turkey, breadcrumbs, egg, parsley, garlic, Worcestershire, fennel seeds, pepper, and salt in a large bowl.

Refrigerate for 10 minutes to firm up. With damp hands, shape the mixture into 32 (1-inch) meatballs (about 1 scant tablespoon each).

- Heat 2 teaspoons oil in a large nonstick skillet over medium heat. Add the meatballs and cook, turning occasionally, until browned on all sides, 7 to 9 minutes. Remove from the heat and add wine, stirring gently to loosen any browned bits.
- To prepare soup: Heat 1 tablespoon oil in a soup pot or Dutch oven over medium heat. Add onion, carrots, and celery and cook, stirring, until the onion is translucent, 7 to 9 minutes. Add cabbage and cook, stirring, 5 minutes more. Stir in broth, beans, escarole (or kale), and the meatballs, and any juice. Bring just to a boil, reduce heat to maintain a simmer, and cook, stirring occasionally, until the vegetables are tender, 20 to 25 minutes. Top each portion with 1 tablespoon grated cheese.

Nutrition

Calories: 284; Protein 23.9g; Carbohydrates 23.5g; Dietary Fiber 6.3g; Sugars 4.6g; Fat 11.1g; Saturated Fat 3.5g; Cholesterol 60.1mg; Vitamin A Iu 4130.1IU; Vitamin C 21.9mg; Folate 141.5mcg; Calcium 205.7mg; Iron 3.3mg; Magnesium 33.3mg; Potassium 869.9mg; Sodium 522.5mg; Thiamin 0.1mg.

4.   Vegan Weight-Loss Lentil Soup

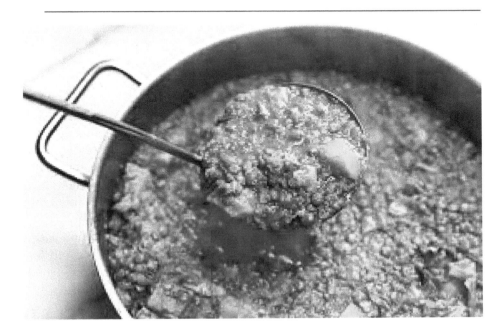

Active: 20 mins

Total: 1 hr

Servings: 6

Ingredients

- 2 tablespoons extra-virgin olive oil
- 1 cup chopped yellow onion
- 1 tablespoon minced garlic
- 2 teaspoons ground turmeric
- 1 teaspoon ground ginger
- ½ teaspoon ground cumin
- 4 cups lower-sodium vegetable broth

- 1 cup dry green lentils
- 1 (15 ounces) can no-salt-added chickpeas, rinsed
- ¾ teaspoon salt
- 1 cup chopped fresh spinach
- 1 cup frozen green beans
- 1 tablespoon fresh lemon juice
- 1 teaspoon crushed red pepper
- Cilantro sprigs for garnish

Instructions

- Heat oil in a medium saucepan over medium heat. Add onion and cook, stirring occasionally, until softened, about 3 minutes. Add garlic, turmeric, ginger, and cumin; cook, stirring constantly, until fragrant, about 1 minute. Stir in broth, lentils, chickpeas, and salt. Bring to a boil over medium-high heat. Reduce heat to medium-low to maintain a simmer; cover and cook, stirring occasionally, until the lentils are tender, 30 to 40 minutes.
- Remove from heat and stir in spinach, green beans, and lemon juice, stirring until the spinach wilts and the green beans are heated for about 1 minute. Ladle the soup into 6 bowls; sprinkle with crushed red pepper and garnish with a sprig of cilantro, if desired.

Nutrition

Calories: 253; Fat 7g; Sodium 479mg; Carbohydrates 37g; Dietary Fiber 9g; Protein 12g; Sugars 4g; Niacin Equivalents 1mg; Saturated Fat 1g; Vitamin A Is 1570IU.

5. Slow-Cooker Mediterranean Chicken & Chickpea Soup

Active: 20 mins

Total: 4 hrs 20 mins

Servings: 6

Ingredients

- 1 ½ cups dried chickpeas, soaked overnight
- 4 cups water
- 1 large yellow onion, finely chopped
- 1 (15 ounces) can no-salt-added diced tomatoes, preferably fire-roasted
- 2 tablespoons tomato paste
- 4 cloves garlic, finely chopped
- 1 bay leaf
- 4 teaspoons ground cumin
- 4 teaspoons paprika
- ¼ teaspoon cayenne pepper
- ¼ teaspoon ground pepper
- 2 pounds bone-in chicken thighs, skin removed, trimmed
- 1 (14 ounces) can artichoke hearts, drained and quartered
- ¼ cup halved pitted oil-cured olives
- ½ teaspoon salt
- ¼ cup chopped fresh parsley or cilantro

Instructions

- Drain chickpeas and place in a 6-quart or larger slow cooker. Add 4 cups water, onion, tomatoes and their juice, tomato paste, garlic, bay leaf, cumin, paprika, cayenne, and ground pepper; stir to combine. Add chicken.

- Cover and cook on Low for 8 hours or High for 4 hours.
- Transfer the chicken to a clean cutting board and let cool slightly. Discard bay leaf. Add artichokes, olives, and salt to the slow cooker and stir to combine. Shred the chicken, discarding bones. Stir the chicken into the soup. Serve topped with parsley (or cilantro).

Nutrition

Calories: 447; Protein 33.6g; Carbohydrates 43g; Dietary Fiber 11.6g; Sugars 8.5g; Fat 15.3g; Saturated Fat 3.3g; Cholesterol 76.5mg; Vitamin A Iu 1590IU; Vitamin C 15.1mg; Folate 194.1mcg; Calcium 114.7mg; Iron 5.7mg; Magnesium 78.7mg; Potassium 608.8mg; Sodium 761.8mg.

6.   Mexican Cabbage Soup

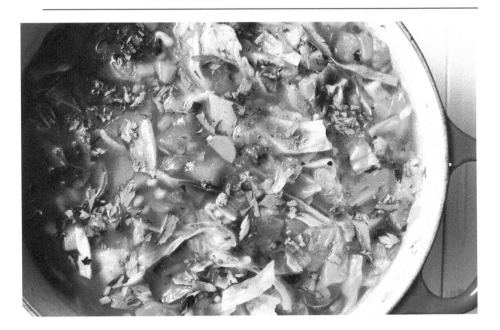

Total: 20 mins

Servings: 8

Ingredient

- 2 tablespoons extra-virgin olive oil
- 2 cups chopped onions
- 1 cup chopped carrot
- 1 cup chopped celery
- 1 cup chopped poblano or green bell pepper
- 4 large cloves garlic, minced
- 8 cups sliced cabbage
- 1 tablespoon tomato paste
- 1 tablespoon minced chipotle chiles in adobo sauce
- 1 teaspoon ground cumin
- ½ teaspoon ground coriander
- 4 cups low-sodium vegetable broth or chicken broth

- 4 cups water
- 2 (15 ounces) cans of low-sodium pinto or black beans, rinsed
- ¾ teaspoon salt
- ½ cup chopped fresh cilantro, plus more for serving
- 2 tablespoons lime juice
- Crumbled queso fresco, nonfat plain Greek yogurt, and/or diced avocado for garnish

Instructions

- Heat oil in a large soup pot (8-quart or larger) over medium heat. Add onions, carrot, celery, poblano (or bell pepper), and garlic; cook, stirring frequently, until softened, 10 to 12 minutes. Add cabbage; cook, stirring occasionally until slightly softened, about 10 minutes more. Add tomato paste, chipotle, cumin, and coriander; cook, stirring, for 1 minute more.
- Add broth, water, beans, and salt. Cover and bring to a boil over high heat. Reduce heat and simmer, partially covered, until the vegetables are tender about 10 minutes. Remove from heat and stir in cilantro and lime juice. Serve garnished with cheese, yogurt, and/or avocado, if desired.

Nutrition

Calories: 167; Protein 6.5g; Carbohydrates 27.1g; Dietary Fiber 8.7g; Sugars 6.6g; Fat 3.8g; Saturated Fat 0.6g; Vitamin A Iu 2968.9IU; Vitamin C 47.2mg; Folate 48.4mcg; Calcium 115mg; Iron 2.3mg; Magnesium 50.5mg; Potassium 623.7mg; Sodium 408.1mg; Thiamin 0.1mg.

7. Roasted Cauliflower & Potato Curry Soup

Active: 50 mins

Total: 1 hr 30 mins

Servings: 8

Ingredients

- 2 teaspoons ground coriander
- 2 teaspoons ground cumin
- 1 ½ teaspoon ground cinnamon
- 1 ½ teaspoon ground turmeric
- 1 ¼ teaspoons salt
- ¾ teaspoon ground pepper
- ⅛ teaspoon cayenne pepper
- 1 small head cauliflower, cut into small florets (about 6 cups)
- 2 tablespoons extra-virgin olive oil, divided
- 1 large onion, chopped
- 1 cup diced carrot
- 3 large cloves garlic, minced
- 1 ½ teaspoons grated fresh ginger
- 1 fresh red chile pepper, such as serrano or jalapeño, minced, plus more for garnish
- 1 (14 ounces) can no-salt-added tomato sauce
- 4 cups low-sodium vegetable broth
- 3 cups diced peeled russet potatoes (1/2-inch)
- 3 cups diced peeled sweet potatoes (1/2-inch)
- 2 teaspoons lime zest
- 2 tablespoons lime juice
- 1 (14 ounces) can coconut milk
- Chopped fresh cilantro for garnish

Instructions

- Preheat oven to 450 degrees F.
- Combine coriander, cumin, cinnamon, turmeric, salt, pepper, and cayenne in a small bowl. Toss cauliflower with 1 tablespoon oil in a large bowl, sprinkle with 1 tablespoon of the spice mixture, and toss again. Spread in a single layer on a rimmed baking sheet. Roast the cauliflower until the edges are browned, 15 to 20 minutes. Set aside.
- Meanwhile, heat the remaining 1 tablespoon oil in a large pot over medium-high heat. Add onion and carrot and cook, stirring often, until starting to brown, 3 to 4 minutes. Reduce heat to medium and continue cooking, stirring often, until the onion is soft, 3 to 4 minutes. Add garlic, ginger, chile, and the remaining spice mixture. Cook, stirring, for 1 minute more.
- Stir in tomato sauce, scraping up any browned bits, and simmer for 1 minute. Add broth, potatoes, sweet potatoes, lime zest, and juice. Cover and bring to a boil over high heat. Reduce heat to maintain a gentle simmer and cook, partially covered and stirring occasionally, until the vegetables are tender, 35 to 40 minutes.
- Stir in coconut milk and the roasted cauliflower. Return to a simmer to heat through. Serve garnished with cilantro and chiles, if desired.

Nutrition

Calories: 272; Protein 5.3g; Carbohydrates 33.4g; Dietary Fiber 7.2g; Sugars 8.3g; Fat 14.8g; Saturated Fat 10.1g; Vitamin A Iu 9200.1IU; Vitamin C 52.2mg; Folate 73.8mcg; Calcium 86.3mg; Iron 3.6mg; Magnesium 69.4mg; Potassium 910.5mg; Sodium 509.4mg.

8.   Turkey & Squash Soup

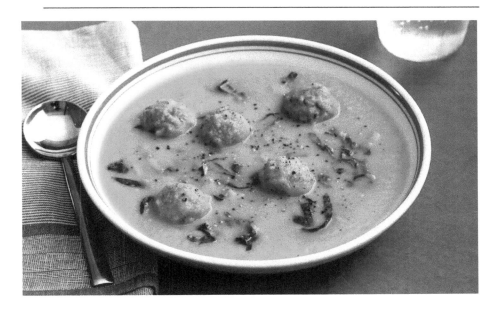

Total: 45 mins

Servings: 6

Ingredients

- 2 teaspoons canola oil
- 2 leeks, trimmed, chopped, and rinsed
- 1 red bell pepper, chopped
- 3 cloves garlic, minced
- 4 cups reduced-sodium chicken broth
- 1 1/2 pounds butternut squash, (1 small to medium), peeled, seeded, and cut into 1-inch cubes
- 2 tablespoons minced fresh thyme, or 2 teaspoons dried thyme
- 1 ½ teaspoon ground cumin
- 1 pound turkey cutlets, cut into 1/2-by-2-inch strips
- 2 cups frozen corn kernels
- 2 tablespoons lime juice
- ½ teaspoon crushed red pepper

- ¼ teaspoon salt
- Freshly ground pepper, to taste

Instructions

- Heat oil in a Dutch oven over medium-high heat. Add leeks and bell pepper; cook, stirring often until the vegetables begin to soften, 3 to 4 minutes. Add garlic and cook, stirring, for 1 minute more. Stir in broth, squash, thyme, and cumin; cover and bring to a boil. Reduce heat to medium-low and cook until the vegetables are tender about 10 minutes.
- Add turkey and corn; return to a simmer and cook until the turkey is just cooked through 3 to 4 minutes. Add lime juice and crushed red pepper. Season with salt and pepper.

Nutrition

Calories: 231; Protein 24.3g; Carbohydrates 31.1g; Dietary Fiber 6.1g; Sugars 6.8g; Fat 2.7g; Saturated Fat 0.2g; Cholesterol 30mg; Vitamin A Iu 12451.7IU; Vitamin C 52mg; Folate 85.5mcg; Calcium 83.8mg; Iron 3.5mg; Magnesium 64.1mg; Potassium 692.2mg; Sodium 550mg; Thiamin 0.1mg.

9.   Baked Vegetable Soup

Total: 1 hr 40 mins

Servings: 8

Ingredients

- 5 tablespoons extra-virgin olive oil
- 1 pound Yukon Gold potatoes, halved and sliced 1/4 inch thick
- 1 ½ teaspoons salt, divided
- 2 medium zucchini, halved and sliced 1/2 inch thick
- 2 medium leeks, white and light green parts only, thinly sliced (see Tip)
- 4 medium stalks celery, thinly sliced
- 10 ounces cremini (Baby Bella) mushrooms, quartered
- 4 cups frozen artichoke hearts (two 9-ounce boxes), thawed, or 10 fresh artichoke hearts, quartered
- ¼ cup chopped fresh parsley, plus more for garnish
- 1 (15 ounces) can no-salt-added diced tomatoes, with their juice
- 1 (2 inches) piece Parmesan cheese rind, plus finely shredded Parmesan for garnish
- 6 cups water
- ½ teaspoon ground pepper

Instructions

- Preheat oven to 350 degrees F.
- Pour oil into a large ovenproof pot (about 6-quart) and arrange potato slices in an even layer over the oil. Sprinkle with 3/4 teaspoon salt. Layer in zucchini, leeks, celery, mushrooms, artichoke hearts, and 1/4 cup parsley; sprinkle with the remaining 3/4 teaspoon salt. Pour tomatoes over the vegetables and nestle Parmesan rind into them. Add water (the vegetables will not be completely submerged), cover, and bring to a boil over high heat.
- Once boiling, transfer the pot to the oven and bake, covered, until the vegetables are tender, but still firm, 1 to 1 1/4 hours. Season with pepper and serve garnished with parsley and Parmesan, if desired.

Nutrition

Calories: 204; Protein 5.2g; Carbohydrates 25.6g; Dietary Fiber 6.9g; Sugars 5.3g; Fat 9.6g; Saturated Fat 1.4g; Vitamin A Iu 1290.4IU; Vitamin C 26.8mg; Folate 148.6mcg; Calcium 97.5mg; Iron 1.7mg; Magnesium 58.4mg; Potassium 812.9mg; Sodium 529.2mg; Thiamin 0.2mg.

10. Slow-Cooker Vegetable Soup

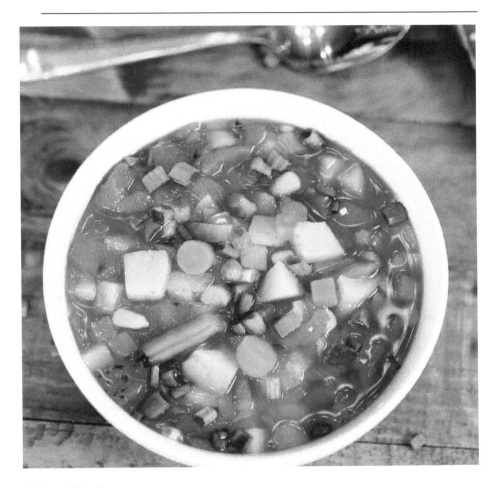

Active: 35 mins

Total: 4 hrs 35 mins

Servings: 8

Ingredients

- 1 medium onion, chopped
- 2 medium carrots, chopped
- 2 stalks celery, chopped
- 12 ounces fresh green beans, cut into 1/2-inch pieces
- 4 cups chopped kale
- 2 medium zucchini, chopped
- 4 Roma tomatoes, seeded and chopped
- 2 cloves garlic, minced
- 2 (15 ounces) cans of no-salt-added cannellini or other white beans, rinsed
- 4 cups low-sodium chicken broth or low-sodium vegetable broth
- 2 teaspoons salt
- ½ teaspoon ground pepper
- 2 teaspoons red-wine vinegar
- 8 teaspoons prepared pesto

Instructions

- Combine onion, carrots, celery, green beans, kale, zucchini, tomatoes, garlic, white beans, broth, salt, and pepper in a 6-quart or larger slow cooker. Cook on High for 4 hours or Low for 6 hours. Stir in vinegar and top each serving of soup with 1 teaspoon pesto.

Nutrition

Calories: 174; Protein 10.3g; Carbohydrates 26.4g; Dietary Fiber 7.6g; Sugars 5.2g; Fat 4.2g; Saturated Fat 0.7g; Vitamin A Iu 4134.1IU; Vitamin C 30.3mg; Folate 52.3mcg; Calcium 101.8mg; Iron 2.8mg; Magnesium 87.4mg; Potassium 762.7mg; Sodium 714.3mg; Thiamin 0.7mg.

11.   311. Butternut Squash Soup With Apple Grilled Cheese Sandwiches

Active: 30 mins

Total: 45 mins

Servings: 4

Ingredient

- 2 tablespoons grapeseed oil or coconut oil, divided
- 1 cup chopped onion
- 2 tablespoons minced fresh ginger
- 1 teaspoon ground cumin
- 1 teaspoon ground turmeric
- ¼ teaspoon cayenne pepper, plus more for garnish
- 5 cups cubed (1-inch) peeled butternut squash
- 1 (15 ounces) can light coconut milk, divided
- 2 cups low-sodium no-chicken broth or chicken broth
- 1 small apple, thinly sliced, divided
- ¾ teaspoon salt
- 1 tablespoon lime juice
- 4 slices whole-wheat country bread
- 1 cup shredded smoked Gouda or Cheddar cheese
- Ground pepper for garnish

Instructions

- Heat 1 tablespoon oil in a large saucepan over medium heat. Add onion and ginger; cook, stirring, until starting to soften, about 3 minutes. Add cumin, turmeric, and cayenne; cook, stirring, for 30 seconds. Add squash, coconut milk (reserve 4 tablespoons for garnish, if desired), broth, half the apple slices, and salt. Bring to a boil. Reduce the heat to maintain a simmer and cook, stirring occasionally, until the squash is tender, about 20 minutes. Stir in lime juice. Remove from heat.

- Puree the soup in the pan using an immersion blender or in batches in a blender. (Use caution when blending hot liquids.)
- Divide 1/2 cup cheese between 2 slices of bread. Top with the remaining apple slices, cheese, and bread. Heat the remaining 1 tablespoon oil in a large nonstick skillet over medium heat. Add the sandwiches and cook until lightly browned on both sides and the cheese is melted, about 2 minutes per side. Cut in half. Garnish the soup with the reserved coconut milk, more cayenne, and ground pepper, if desired.

Nutrition

Calories: 419; Protein 13.5g; Carbohydrates 43.3g; Dietary Fiber 8.4g; Sugars 10.4g; Fat 23.1g; Saturated Fat 10.6g; Cholesterol 26.3mg; Vitamin A Iu 16927.8IU; Vitamin C 28.5mg; Folate 49.7mcg; Calcium 298.2mg; Iron 2.2mg; Magnesium 72.9mg; Potassium 622.5mg; Sodium 826.9mg.

12. Winter Minestrone

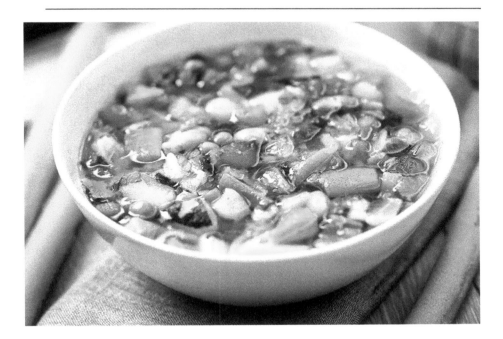

Active: 40 mins

Total: 4 hrs 45 mins

Servings: 8

Ingredient

- 1 pound uncooked Italian or pork sausage links, cut into 3/4-inch slices
- 2 ½ cups peeled winter squash, such as butternut squash, cut into 1-inch cubes
- 1 ½ cups cubed potatoes
- 2 medium fennel bulbs, trimmed and cut into 1-inch pieces
- 1 large onion, chopped
- 2 cloves garlic, minced
- 1 (15 ounces) can of red kidney beans, rinsed and drained

- ½ teaspoon dried sage, crushed
- 4 cups chicken broth or vegetable broth
- 1 cup dry white wine
- 4 cups chopped kale or fresh spinach

Instructions

- In a large skillet, cook the sausage until browned; drain well.
- In a 5- to the 6-quart slow cooker, place squash, potatoes, fennel, onion, garlic, beans, and sage. Top with sausage. Pour broth and wine overall.
- Cover and cook on Low for 8 to 10 hours or on High for 4 to 5 hours. Stir in kale (or spinach). Cover and cook 5 minutes more.

Nutrition

Calories: 315; Protein 16g; Carbohydrates 27g; Dietary Fiber 14g; Sugars 1g; Fat 14g; Saturated Fat 5g; Cholesterol 38mg; Sodium 933mg.

13. Garden-Fresh Asparagus Soup

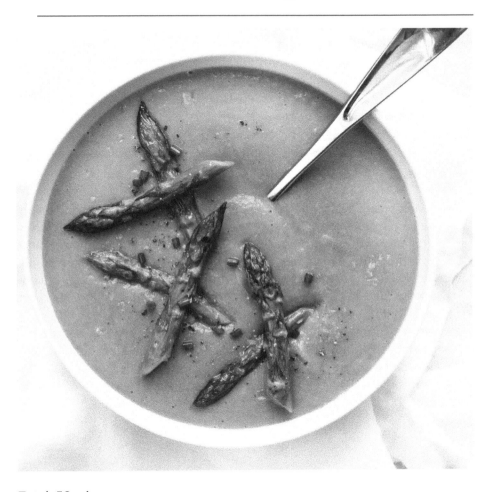

Total: 50 mins

Servings: 6

Ingredient

- 2 tablespoons butter

- 2 tablespoons extra-virgin olive oil
- 1 medium onion, finely chopped
- ½ teaspoon salt
- ½ teaspoon curry powder
- ¼ teaspoon ground ginger
- Zest and juice of 1 lemon, divided
- 2 cups diced peeled red potatoes
- 3 cups vegetable broth, or reduced-sodium chicken broth
- 1 cup "lite" coconut milk
- 2 cups 1/2-inch pieces trimmed asparagus, (about 1 bunch)
- Freshly ground pepper to taste
- ¼ cup crème fraîche or reduced-fat sour cream
- 1/4 cup finely chopped scallion greens, or fresh chives

Instructions

- Melt butter and oil in a large saucepan over medium heat. Add onion and 1/4 teaspoon salt and cook, stirring often, until golden, about 5 minutes. Stir in curry powder, ginger, lemon zest, and potatoes and simmer, stirring occasionally, for 5 minutes. Stir in broth, coconut milk, and asparagus. Bring to a simmer over medium heat, partially cover, and continue to cook until
- The potatoes are tender, about 15 minutes.
- Puree the soup with an immersion blender or a regular blender (in batches) until smooth. (Use caution when pureeing hot liquids.) Season with the remaining 1/4 teaspoon salt and pepper.
- Whisk creme fraiche (or sour cream), lemon juice, and scallion greens (or chives) in a small bowl and garnish with a swirl of it.

Nutrition

Calories: 181; Protein 5.2g; Carbohydrates 15.1g; Dietary Fiber 2.3g; Sugars 2.6g; Fat 12.1g; Saturated Fat 5.3g; Cholesterol 10.2mg; Vitamin C 13.8mg; Folate 35.8mcg; Calcium 28.7mg; Iron 1.6mg; Magnesium 21.2mg; Potassium 455.9mg; Sodium 251.1mg; Thiamin 0.1mg.

14. Creamy Chopped Cauliflower Salad

Total: 15 mins

Servings: 6

Ingredients

- 5 tablespoons reduced-fat mayonnaise
- 2 tablespoons cider vinegar
- 1 small shallot, finely chopped
- 1/2 teaspoon caraway seeds, (optional)
- ¼ teaspoon freshly ground pepper
- 3 cups chopped cauliflower florets, (about 1/2 large head)
- 2 cups chopped heart of romaine
- 1 tart-sweet red apple, chopped

Instructions

- Whisk mayonnaise, vinegar, shallot, caraway seeds (if using), and pepper in a large bowl until smooth. Add cauliflower, romaine, and apple; toss to coat.

Nutrition

Calories: 68; Protein 1.5g; Carbohydrates 10.9g; Dietary Fiber 2.2g; Sugars 5.1g; Fat 2.6g; Saturated Fat 0.4g; Cholesterol 3.1mg; Vitamin A Iu 1437.8IU; Vitamin C 29.5mg; Folate 56.1mcg; Calcium 22.9mg; Iron 0.5mg; Magnesium 13.4mg; Potassium 256.8mg; Sodium 120.3mg; Thiamin 0.1mg.

15. Spinach & Warm Mushroom Salad

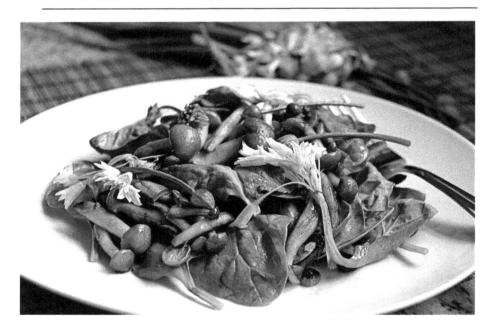

Total: 30 mins

Servings: 4

Ingredients

- 8 cups spinach, tough stems removed
- 2 cups coarsely chopped radicchio
- 2 tablespoons extra-virgin olive oil, divided
- 2 slices bacon, chopped
- 1 large shallot, halved and sliced (1/2 cup)
- 3 cups sliced mixed mushrooms, such as shiitake, oyster, and cremini
- ¼ teaspoon salt
- ¼ teaspoon ground pepper
- 2 tablespoons white balsamic vinegar

- ½ teaspoon honey

Instructions

- Combine spinach and radicchio in a large bowl.
- Heat 1 tablespoon oil in a large skillet over medium heat. Add bacon and shallot and cook, stirring, until the bacon is crisp, 4 to 5 minutes. Add mushrooms, salt, and pepper and cook, stirring, until the mushrooms are tender, 5 to 7 minutes. Remove from heat and stir in the remaining 1 tablespoon oil, vinegar, and honey, scraping up any browned bits. Immediately pour the warm vinaigrette over the spinach mixture and toss to coat.

Nutrition

Calories; Protein 4.7g; Carbohydrates 11.5g; Dietary Fiber 2.7g; Sugars 3.9g; Fat 8.8g; Saturated Fat 1.5g; Cholesterol 3.5mg; Vitamin A Iu 5871.6IU; Vitamin C 20.1mg; Folate 140.7mcg; Calcium 74.7mg; Iron 2.3mg; Magnesium 64.8mg; Potassium 617.8mg; Sodium 259.6mg; Thiamin 0.1mg; Added Sugar 1g.

16.   Fattoush

Total: 40 mins

Servings: 8

Ingredients

- 2 6-inch whole-wheat pitas, split
- 3 tablespoons extra-virgin olive oil, divided
- 1 1/4 teaspoons ground sumac, (see note), divided
- ¼ cup lemon juice
- ½ teaspoon salt
- ¼ teaspoon freshly ground pepper
- 1 large head of romaine lettuce, coarsely chopped
- 2 large tomatoes, diced
- 2 small salad cucumbers, or 1 large cucumber, seeded and diced
- ½ cup thinly sliced red onion
- ⅓ cup thinly sliced fresh mint

Instructions

- Preheat oven to 350F.
- Place pita halves rough-side up on a large baking sheet. Brush with 1 tablespoon oil and sprinkle with 1 teaspoon sumac. Bake until the pita halves are golden and crisp, about 15 minutes. When cool, break into bite-size pieces.
- Whisk lemon juice, salt, pepper, and the remaining 2 tablespoons oil and 1/4 teaspoon sumac in a large bowl. Add lettuce, tomatoes, cucumber, onion, mint, and the pita pieces;
- Toss to coat. Let stand for 15 minutes before serving.

Nutrition

Calories: 117; Protein 2.9g; Carbohydrates 14.9g; Dietary Fiber 3.2g; Sugars 2.9g; Fat 6g; Saturated Fat 0.9g; Vitamin A Iu 3820.9IU; Vitamin C 12.7mg; Folate 70.1mcg; Calcium 35.5mg; Iron 1.6mg;

Magnesium 30.2mg; Potassium 322.3mg; Sodium 224mg; Thiamin 0.1mg.

17. Mixed Green Salad With Grapefruit & Cranberries

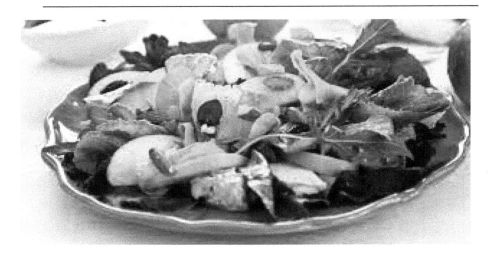

Total: 25 mins

Servings:12

Ingredients

- 2 red grapefruit
- ¼ cup extra-virgin olive oil
- 2 tablespoons minced scallions
- 1 tablespoon white-wine vinegar
- ¼ teaspoon salt
- ¼ teaspoon freshly ground pepper
- 8 cups torn butter lettuce
- 6 cups baby spinach
- 1 14-ounce can hearts of palm (see Shopping Tip), drained and cut into bite-size pieces
- ⅓ cup dried cranberries
- 1/3 cup toasted pine nuts

Instructions

- Remove the skin and white pith from grapefruit with a sharp knife. Working over a bowl, cut the segments from their surrounding membranes. Cut the segments in half on a cutting board and transfer to a large salad bowl. Squeeze the grapefruit peel and membranes over the original bowl to extract 1/4 cup grapefruit juice.
- Whisk oil, scallions, vinegar, salt, and pepper into the bowl with the grapefruit juice.
- Add lettuce, spinach, and hearts of palm to the salad bowl with the grapefruit segments. Just before serving, toss the salad with the dressing until well coated. Sprinkle cranberries and pine nuts on top.

Nutrition

Calories: 162; Protein 3.3g; Carbohydrates 14.9g; Dietary Fiber 3.2g; Sugars 8.4g; Fat 11.3g; Saturated Fat 1.3g; Vitamin A Iu 4656.3IU; Vitamin C 30mg; Folate 104.9mcg; Calcium 72.7mg; Iron 2.5mg; Magnesium 55mg; Potassium 424.8mg; Sodium 205.3mg; Thiamin 0.1mg; Added Sugar 3g.

18. Melon, Tomato & Onion Salad With Goat Cheese

Total: 30 mins

Servings: 8

Ingredient

- 1 cup very thinly sliced sweet white onion, separated into rings
- 1 small firm-ripe melon
- 2 large tomatoes, very thinly sliced
- 1 small cucumber, very thinly sliced
- ½ teaspoon kosher salt
- ¼ teaspoon freshly ground pepper
- 1 cup crumbled goat cheese
- ¼ cup extra-virgin olive oil
- 4 teaspoons balsamic vinegar
- ⅓ cup very thinly sliced fresh basil

Instructions

- Place onion rings in a medium bowl, add cold water to cover and a handful of ice cubes. Set aside for about 20 minutes. Drain and pat dry.
- Meanwhile, cut melon in half lengthwise and scoop out the seeds. Remove the rind with a sharp knife. Place each melon half cut-side down and slice crosswise into 1/8-inch-thick slices.
- Make the salad on a large platter or 8 individual salad plates. Begin by arranging a ring of melon slices around the edge. Top with a layer of overlapping tomato slices. Arrange a second ring of melon slices toward the center. Top with the remaining tomato slices. Tuck cucumber slices between the layers of tomato and melon. Sprinkle with salt and pepper. Top with goat cheese and the onion rings. Drizzle with oil and vinegar. Sprinkle with basil.

Nutrition

Calories: 194; Protein 4.7g; Carbohydrates 19.4g; Dietary Fiber 2.3g; Sugars 16g; Fat 11.6g; Saturated Fat 4g; Cholesterol 11.2mg; Vitamin A Iu 774.7IU; Vitamin C 37.5mg; Folate 45.3mcg; Calcium 67.2mg; Iron 0.8mg; Magnesium 30.7mg; Potassium 570.6mg; Sodium 161.2mg; Thiamin 0.1mg.

19. Curried Carrot Soup

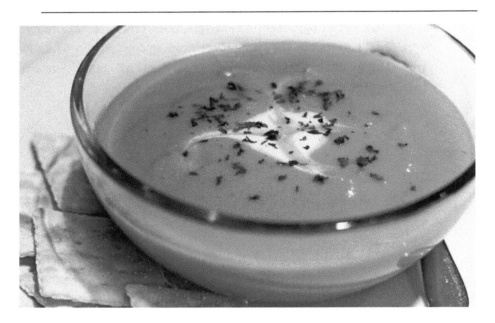

Total: 1 hr

Servings: 6

Ingredients

- 3 tablespoons canola oil
- 2 teaspoons curry powder
- 8 medium carrots, peeled and thinly sliced
- 4 medium stalks celery, thinly sliced
- 1 medium onion, coarsely chopped
- 5 cups reduced-sodium chicken broth
- 1 tablespoon lemon juice
- ½ teaspoon salt
- Freshly ground pepper, to taste

Instructions

- Cook oil and curry powder in a large saucepan over medium heat, stirring, until fragrant, 1 to 2 minutes. Stir in carrots, celery, and onion; toss to coat in oil. Cook, stirring frequently, for 10 minutes. Stir in broth. Bring to a boil. Reduce heat and simmer until the vegetables are very tender about 10 minutes. Remove from the heat; let stand 10 minutes. Lay a paper towel over the surface of the soup to blot away the oil that has risen to the top. Discard the paper towel.
- Working in batches of no more than 2 cups at a time, transfer the soup to a blender and puree (use caution when pureeing hot liquids). Return the pureed soup to the pan, place over medium heat, and heat through. Season with lemon juice, salt, and pepper.

Nutrition

Calories: 122; Protein 4g; Carbohydrates 11.7g; Dietary Fiber 3.4g; Sugars 5.5g; Fat 7.4g; Saturated Fat 0.6g; Vitamin A Iu 13708.5IU; Vitamin C 8.8mg; Folate 35.4mcg; Calcium 45.9mg; Iron 0.7mg; Magnesium 18.5mg; Potassium 538.1mg; Sodium 637.5mg; Thiamin 0.1mg.

20. Clam Chowder

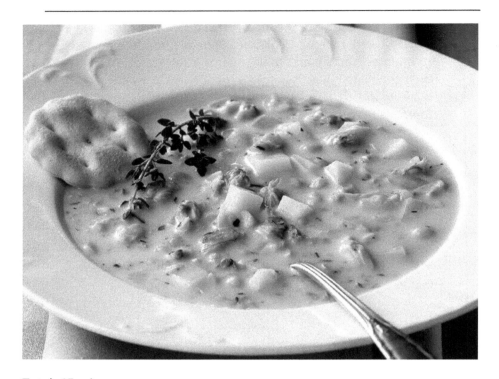

Total: 45 mins

Servings: 6

Ingredients

- 3 tablespoons extra-virgin olive oil
- 1 cup diced onion
- 1 cup diced celery
- ½ cup all-purpose flour
- ½ teaspoon dried thyme
- ¼ teaspoon salt
- ¼ teaspoon ground pepper
- 1 bay leaf
- 4 cups clam juice (see Tip) or seafood stock

- 1 cup whole milk
- 3 cups diced white potatoes
- 1 16-ounce container chopped fresh clams (plus their liquid), thawed if frozen
- Chopped cooked bacon for garnish
- Snipped chives for garnish

Instructions

- Heat oil in a large pot over medium heat. Add onion and celery; cook, stirring frequently until softened and beginning to brown, 3 to 6 minutes. Sprinkle flour, thyme, salt, pepper, and bay leaf over the vegetables and cook, stirring, for 1 minute more. Add clam juice (or seafood stock) and milk; bring to a gentle boil, stirring constantly.
- Stir in potatoes and bring just to a simmer. Simmer, uncovered, stirring occasionally, until the potatoes are tender, 12 to 15 minutes.
- Add clams and cook, stirring frequently, until cooked through, 2 to 4 minutes. Serve topped with bacon and chives, if desired.

Nutrition

Calories: 229; Protein 12.2g; Carbohydrates 26.5g; Dietary Fiber 3.6g; Sugars 5g; Fat 9g; Saturated Fat 1.8g; Cholesterol 35.3mg; Folate 60.4mcg; Calcium 105.1mg; Iron 2.9mg; Magnesium 44.6mg; Potassium 693.2mg; Sodium 476.8mg; Thiamin 0.2mg.

21. New Mexico Chile Verde (Green Chili)

Prep Time: 30 Minutes

Cook Time: 3 Hours 30 Minutes

Total Time: 4 Hours

Ingredients

- 1/4 cup oil
- 4 pounds pork butt, trimmed and cut into 1 1/2-inch cube
- 2 large onions, peeled and chopped
- 1 tablespoon ground cumin
- 1 tablespoon ground coriander
- 1 tablespoon oregano
- 4 cloves garlic, minced
- 2 Hatch peppers, chopped (or Anaheims)
- 2 Poblano peppers, chopped
- 1-2 jalapeno peppers, seeded and diced
- 1 pound tomatillos (peeled and cleaned), chopped
- 2 bay leaves
- 1 bunch cilantro (large), chopped
- 3 tablespoons masa (corn flour)
- 4 cups water or chicken stock
- 1 tablespoon salt, divided
- Lime wedges for garnish

Instructions

- Heat the oil in a large pot over medium-high heat. Add the pork and 2 teaspoons of salt. Brown the pork on all sides, stirring regularly.

Remove the pork from the pot and pour out all rendered fat, saving about 1 tablespoon.

- Add the onions, remaining salt, cumin, coriander, and oregano to the pot. Sauté for 3-5 minutes. Then add the garlic and peppers. Sauté another 3-5 minutes. Add the chopped tomatillos, bay leaves, and cilantro. Toss the pork with the masa and add back to the pot. Stir well.
- Finally, add the water. Bring to a boil, then reduce the heat to low. Cover and simmer for 3 hours, or until the pork is falling apart, stirring occasionally.
- Take 2 forks and break the pork up even more. Salt and pepper to taste.

Nutrition

Serving: 1cup, Calories: 626kcal, Carbohydrates: 23g, Protein: 63g, Fat: 30g, Saturatedfat: 7g, Cholesterol: 186mg, Sodium: 1657mg, Potassium: 1599mg, Fiber: 5g, Sugar: 8g, Vitamin C: 49.9mg, Calcium: 115mg, Iron: 6.4mg

22. Pozole Verde De Pollo (Chicken Pozole)

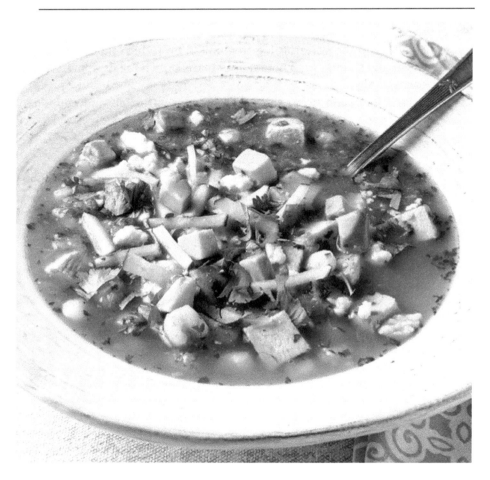

Prep Time: 15 Minutes

Cook Time: 1 Hour 10 Minutes

Total Time: 1 Hour 25 Minutes

Servings: 8 Servings

Ingredients

- 2 tablespoons olive oil
- 1 large sweet onion peeled and chopped
- 6-8 cloves garlic minced
- 6 poblano peppers seeded and chopped
- 2-3 jalapeno peppers seeded and chopped (optional for heat)
- ½ cup chopped cilantro
- 3 pounds boneless chicken thighs
- 1 ½ pounds tomatillos peeled and quartered
- 2 bay leaves
- 1 tablespoon dried oregano
- 6 cups chicken broth or water
- 2 – 15 ounce cans white hominy drained and rinsed
- Salt and pepper
- Garnishes: Tortilla chips, shredded cabbage, lime wedges, sliced avocado, sliced radishes, chopped cilantro

Instructions

- Set a heavy 6-8 quart dutch oven over medium heat. Add the oil to the pot. Add in the chopped onion and garlic. Sauté for 2 minutes, then add in the chopped poblanos, jalapenos, and cilantro. Sauté another 8 minutes, stirring regularly.
- Place the chicken thighs, tomatillos, bay leaves, oregano, chicken broth, and 1 teaspoon salt.
- Cover the pot with a heavy lid and bring to a boil. Then lower the heat and simmer for 50-60 minutes, until the chicken is soft enough to shred. (Keep the pot covered.)
- Remove the chicken thighs, and bay leaves. Use tongs or forks to shred the chicken into small chunks.
- Add the shredded chicken back to the pot, along with the rinsed hominy. Stir to combine. Simmer another 2-3 minutes to warm the hominy. Taste, then season with salt and pepper as needed. Keep warm until ready to serve.
- To Serve: Ladle the posole into bowls. Garnish the top with tortilla chips, shredded cabbage, sliced avocado, radishes, lime wedges, and cilantro.

Nutrition

Calories: 477kcal, Carbohydrates: 15g, Protein: 31g, Fat: 33g, Saturatedfat: 8g, Cholesterol: 167mg, Sodium: 785mg, Potassium: 954mg, Fiber: 4g, Sugar: 8g, Vitamin A: 676iu, Vitamin C: 101mg, Calcium: 61mg, Iron: 3mg

23. The Ultimate Wedge Salad Recipe

Prep Time: 15 Minutes

Cook Time: 5 Minutes

Total Time: 20 Minutes

Servings: 4 Servings

Ingredients

For The Blue Cheese Dressing:

- ½ cup sour cream
- ½ cup mayonnaise
- 1/3 cup buttermilk
- 1 tablespoon apple cider vinegar
- ½ teaspoon salt
- ¼ teaspoon cracked black pepper
- ¼ teaspoon garlic powder
- ½ cup crumbled blue cheese

For The Wedge Salad:

- 8 slices bacon chopped
- 1 head iceberg lettuce
- 1 cup cherry or grape tomatoes halved
- 1 cup blue cheese dressing
- ½ cup chopped scallions
- ½ cup crumbled blue cheese

Instructions

Make The Dressing: Set out a medium mixing bowl. Add the sour cream, mayonnaise, buttermilk, apple cider vinegar, salt, pepper, and garlic powder.

Stir well. Then mix in the crumbled blue cheese. Cover and chill until ready to use. (If possible, make a day ahead, or early in the day, so the blue cheese has time to permeate the dressing.)

Cook The Bacon: Set a skillet over medium heat. Place the chopped bacon in the skillet. Brown the bacon for 4-6 minutes until crispy, stirring regularly. Then scoop the bacon out of the skillet onto a paper towel-lined plate to drain off the grease.

Prep The Veggies: Slice the tomatoes in half and chop the scallions. Then set the head of lettuce on the cutting board. Trim the root/core end a little. Cut the head in half, through the core. (This helps hold the wedges together.) Then cut each half in two, through the core.

Stack The Wedges: Set each lettuce wedge on a plate. Drizzle with a generous amount of blue cheese dressing. (At least ¼ cup per salad.) Then sprinkle the tops with halved tomatoes, scallions, bacon, and more blue cheese crumbles. Finish each salad plate off with a bit of fresh cracked pepper. Serve cold.

Nutrition

Calories: 653kcal, Carbohydrates: 12g, Protein: 19g, Fat: 59g, Saturatedfat: 21g, Cholesterol: 84mg, Sodium: 1870mg, Potassium: 547mg, Fiber: 2g, Sugar: 8g, Vitamin C: 15mg, Calcium: 325mg, Iron: 2mg

24. Crispy Brussel Sprouts Quinoa Salad Recipe

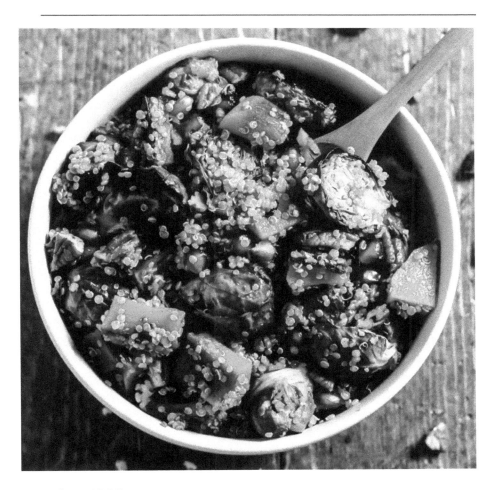

Prep Time: 15 Minutes

Cook Time: 30 Minutes

Total Time: 45 Minutes

Servings: 8

Ingredients

- 1 1/4 cup dried lentils, choose a more firm lentil type
- 2/3 cup dried quinoa
- 3 cups water
- 3/4 teaspoon curry powder
- 8 ounces Brussels sprouts
- 1 cup thinly sliced shallots, about 3-4
- 2 tablespoons olive oil
- 1/2 cup DeLallo Sun-Dried Peppers, chopped
- 1/2 cup scallions, chopped
- 1/2 lemon, juiced
- Salt and pepper

Instructions

- Preheat the oven to 400 degrees F. Place the quinoa and lentils in a medium stockpot with 3 cups of water, 1 teaspoon salt, and 3/4 teaspoon curry powder. Bring to a boil, then cover and reduce the heat to medium-low. Cook for 25-30 minutes until the quinoa is fluffy and the lentils are cooked, but firm. Remove from heat, but keep covered until ready to use.
- Meanwhile, cut the Brussels sprouts in half and slice thin. Place them on a rimmed baking sheet with the sliced shallots and drizzle with olive oil. Toss to coat then spread them out thin and salt and pepper. Bake for 20-25 minutes, until crispy.
- Fluff the quinoa and lentils and move to a large bowl. Add the crispy Brussels sprouts and shallots, chopped sweet peppers, chopped scallions, and the juice of half a lemon. Toss and salt and pepper to taste. Serve immediately.

Nutrition

Calories: 214kcal, Carbohydrates: 33g, Protein: 11g, Fat: 5g, Saturatedfat: 1g, Sodium: 18mg, Potassium: 546mg, Fiber: 12g, Sugar: 3g, Vitamin A: 900iu, Vitamin C: 30.9mg, Calcium: 44mg, Iron: 3.6mg

25. Hungarian Mushroom Soup (Vegan or Gluten-Free!)

Prep Time: 10 Minutes

Cook Time: 33 Minutes

Total Time: 43 Minutes

Servings: 6 Servings

Ingredients

- ¼ cups butter (or plant-based butter)
- 1 large onion peeled and chopped
- 1 cup chopped celery
- 1 pound button mushrooms sliced
- 3 tablespoons soy sauce (gluten-free)
- 2 tablespoons fresh chopped dill
- 1 tablespoon smoked paprika
- 1 tablespoon lemon juice
- 6 cups vegetable broth or mushroom broth
- ¾ cups sour cream (or Vegan Cashew Sour Cream)
- 3 tablespoons all-purpose flour (or GF baking mix)
- Salt and pepper
- Garnishes: Fresh chopped dill, scallions, and/or parsley, sour cream, or cashew cream

Instructions

- Set a large 6-quart saucepot over medium heat. Add the butter, onions, and celery. Sauté for 3-5 minutes to soften. Then move the veggies to the side of the pot and add in the mushrooms, 1 teaspoon salt, and ½ teaspoon pepper. Sauté another 8-10 minutes, stirring regularly.
- Stir in the soy sauce, dill, smoked paprika, lemon juice, and vegetable broth. Simmer for 10-15 minutes.

- Meanwhile, set out a medium bowl. Add the sour cream and flour. Stir until smooth.
- Ladle some of the soup broth into the sour cream mixture, stirring constantly so the sour cream doesn't curdle. Once the mixture is thin, whisk the sour cream mixture into the soup base, whisking continually.
- Simmer another 3-5 minutes to thicken. Taste, then add additional salt and lemon juice if needed.
- Serve warm with a sprinkling of fresh herbs and a dollop of sour cream on top.

Nutrition

Calories: 185kcal, Carbohydrates: 13g, Protein: 5g, Fat: 14g, Saturatedfat: 8g, Cholesterol: 35mg, Sodium: 1552mg, Potassium: 397mg, Fiber: 2g, Sugar: 6g, Vitamin A: 1577iu, Vitamin C: 5mg, Calcium: 52mg, Iron: 1mg

26.   Zesty Wor Wonton Soup Recipe

Prep Time: 35 Minutes

Cook Time: 15 Minutes

Total Time: 50 Minutes

Servings: 8 Servings

Ingredients

For The Wontons:

- ½ pound ground pork or chicken
- ¼ cup chopped scallions
- 2 tablespoons soy sauce
- 2-3 cloves garlic minced
- 1 tablespoon fresh grated ginger
- 1 teaspoon sesame oil
- ½ teaspoon crushed red pepper
- 25 refrigerated wontons wrappers usually 2-inch squares

For The Wonton Soup:

- 1 tablespoon sesame oil
- 3-4 cloves garlic minced
- 1 tablespoon fresh grated ginger
- 8 cups chicken broth
- 2 tablespoons soy sauce
- 2 cups cooked shredded chicken use up leftovers
- 2 cups chopped bok choy
- 8 ounces sliced shiitake mushrooms
- ½ cup chopped scallions

Instructions

For The Wontons:

- Set out a medium mixing bowl. Add ground pork or chicken, scallions, soy sauce, garlic, ginger, sesame oil, and crushed red pepper. Mix until well combined.
- Layout several wontons wrappers. Set out a small dish of water to act as glue. Place 1 ½ teaspoon of the meat filling in the center of each wonton. Use your finger to paint a line of water along two connected edges. Fold the wet corner up to meet the opposite corner. Use your fingers to close and seal the edges of the wonton wrapper, making a triangle shape.
- Now use your finger to dampen the two bottom corners. Bring them together and pinch to seal. Repeat with the remaining wonton wrappers and filling.

For The Wonton Soup:

- Set a large 6-8 quart saucepot over medium-high heat. Add the sesame oil, garlic, and ginger. Sauté for 2 minutes, to soften the aromatics, then pour in the chicken broth and soy sauce. Bring to a simmer. Simmer the soup base for 10 minutes.
- Meanwhile, load soup bowls with shredded chicken, bok choy, sliced mushrooms, and scallions. (These ingredients will steep in the hot broth, "Hot Pot" style!)
- Once the soup has simmered 10 minutes, reduce the heat, and gently lower the wontons into the soup. Simmer on medium-low for 2-3 minutes. (DO NOT over-cook the wontons or they will open up and disintegrate into the soup.) Then ladle the wonton soup broth into the bowls. Serve hot.

Nutrition

Calories: 165kcal, Carbohydrates: 19g, Protein: 10g, Fat: 6g, Saturatedfat: 1g, Cholesterol: 26mg, Sodium: 1532mg, Potassium: 535mg, Fiber: 2g, Sugar: 1g, Vitamin A: 912iu, Vitamin C: 27mg, Calcium: 55mg, Iron: 2mg

27. Creamy Parmesan Chicken And Rice Soup

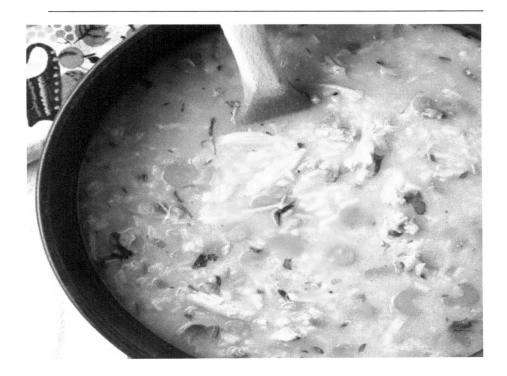

Prep Time: 15 Minutes

Cook Time: 30 Minutes

Total Time: 45 Minutes

Servings: 8 People

Ingredients

- 2 tablespoons butter
- 1 large sweet onion, peeled and chopped
- 1 cup chopped carrots

- 1 cup chopped celery
- 4 cloves garlic, minced
- 1 tablespoon fresh thyme leaves, 1 tsp dried thyme
- 1 bay leaf
- 1 pound boneless chicken thighs, or breasts
- 10 cups chicken broth, or water + 10 tsp chicken bouillon
- 1 cup dried long-grain rice
- 2/3 cup grated parmesan cheese
- 3 tablespoons cornstarch
- 3 tablespoons chopped parsley
- Salt and pepper

Instructions

- Place a large 6-8 quart pot over medium heat. Add the butter. Once melted add in the onions, carrots, celery, and garlic. Sauté for 3-5 minutes, stirring to soften.
- Add in the thyme, bay leaf, chicken thighs, and chicken broth. Bring to a boil. Once boiling, stir in the dried rice.
- Cover and simmer for 12 minutes. Then use tongs to remove the chicken thighs. Use two forks to shred the chicken into bite-size pieces. Continue to simmer the soup uncovered, while you shred the chicken.
- Mix the grated parmesan cheese with the cornstarch. Stir the chicken back into the soup. Continue stirring as you add the parmesan mixture into the soup. Simmer another 2-4 minutes to thicken the soup base.
- Taste. Then salt and pepper as needed. Remove the bay leaf and stir in the fresh parsley. Serve warm.

Nutrition

Calories: 321kcal, Carbohydrates: 29g, Protein: 16g, Fat: 16g,Saturatedfat: 6g, Cholesterol: 70mg, Sodium: 1298mg, Potassium: 541mg, Fiber: 2g, Sugar: 3g, Vitamin C: 28mg, Calcium: 148mg, Iron: 2mg

28. Nana's Epic Navy Bean Ham Bone Soup

Prep Time: 10 Minutes

Cook Time: 1 Hour 10 Minutes

Total Time: 1 Hour 20 Minutes

Servings: 8

Ingredients

- 1 pound dried navy beans
- 1 ham bone + ham scraps
- 1 tablespoon olive oil
- 1 large onion, peeled and chopped
- 6 cloves garlic, minced
- 1 tablespoon fresh thyme leaves
- 2 teaspoons ground cumin
- 1/2-1 teaspoon crushed red pepper
- 10 cups water
- Salt and pepper

Instructions

- The Night Before: Place the dried beans in a large bowl and cover with three inches of water. Soak the dried beans overnight (up to 24 hours) to soften. Drain when ready to use.
- Place a large 6-quart pot over medium heat. Add the oil, ham bone, onions, and garlic. Sauté for 3-5 minutes to soften the onions.
- Then add in the drained beans, thyme, ground cumin, crushed red pepper, 10 cups of water, and any remaining ham scraps. (Do not salt the soup until the end, because ham bones can be very salty.)
- Bring the soup to a boil. Lower the heat and simmer for 60-90 minutes, covered, until the beans are very soft. Uncover and stir occasionally, then place the lid back on top.

- Use a fork to pull any remaining ham off the bone and stir it into the soup. Discard the bone. Add 1-2 cups additional water if the soup is too thick. Taste, then salt and pepper as needed.

Nutrition

Calories: 218kcal, Carbohydrates: 36g, Protein: 13g, Fat: 2g, Saturatedfat: 0g, Cholesterol: 0mg, Sodium: 22mg, Potassium: 715mg, Fiber: 14g, Sugar: 2g, Vitamin A: 85iu, Vitamin C: 3.1mg, Calcium: 108mg, Iron: 3.7mg

29.   Turkey Chili

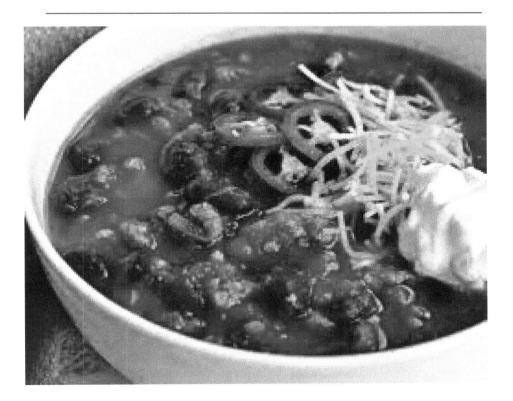

Prep Time: 15 Minutes

Cook Time: 30 Minutes

Total Time: 45 Minutes

Servings: 6

Ingredients

- 1 1/2 cup red bell pepper, diced
- 1 cup red onion, diced
- 1 cup celery, chopped
- 4 cloves garlic, minced

- 1/2 cup butter
- 6 tablespoons masa (corn flour)
- 2 tablespoons ground cumin
- 2 tablespoons ground coriander
- 1 1/2 tablespoons chili powder
- 1 tablespoon dried oregano
- 6 cups turkey stock or chicken stock
- 6 cups turkey meat, cooked and chopped
- 45 ounces canned black beans, drained and rinsed
- 1 1/2 cups frozen corn
- 2 tablespoon honey
- Salt and pepper to taste
- Possible Toppings: shredded cheese, sour cream, diced red onion, chopped scallions, salsa, corn chips

Instructions

- Place the butter in a large stockpot and set over medium heat. Add the bell pepper, onions, celery, and garlic. Sauté for 5-8 minutes, until softened. Stir to make sure the veggies don't burn.
- Mix in the masa, cumin, coriander, chili powder, and oregano. Stir to coat and sauté for another 2 minutes. Then pour in the turkey stock and scrape the bottom of the pot to loosen the veggies.
- Add the chopped turkey, beans, corn, and honey. Season with 1 1/2 teaspoons of salt and 1/2 teaspoon ground pepper. Bring the chili to a low boil and simmer for at least 20 minutes, stirring occasionally. Taste and season again if needed. Serve warm.

Nutrition

Calories: 674kcal, Carbohydrates: 37g, Protein: 95g, Fat: 16g, Saturatedfat: 6g, Cholesterol: 234mg, Sodium: 1476mg, Potassium: 1607mg, Fiber: 9g, Sugar: 6g, Vitamin C: 30.2mg, Calcium: 139mg, Iron: 6.2mg

30. Classic Beef Barley Soup

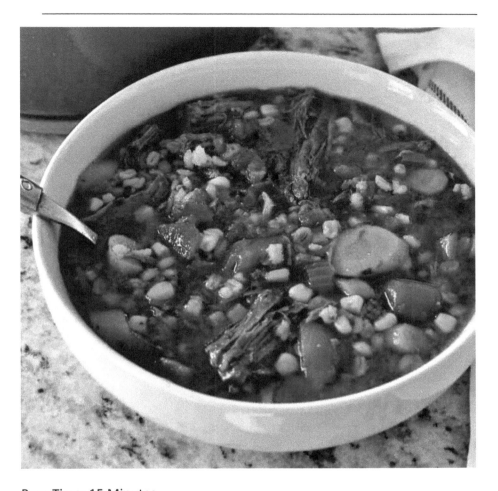

Prep Time: 15 Minutes

Cook Time: 45 Minutes

Total Time: 1 Hour

Servings: 8 Servings

Ingredients

- 1 tablespoon olive oil
- 2 1/2 - 3 pounds beef chuck roast
- 1 large sweet onion, peeled and chopped
- 2 cups sliced carrots
- 2 cups sliced celery
- 4 cloves garlic, minced
- 12 cups beef broth
- 15 ounces fire-roasted diced tomatoes (1 can)
- 1 cup dried barley
- 1 tablespoon fresh thyme leaves (1 teaspoon dried)
- 1 tablespoon freshly chopped rosemary leaves (1 teaspoon dried)
- 1/2 teaspoon crushed red pepper
- Salt and pepper

Instructions

- Place a large saucepot over medium heat and add the olive oil and onions. Saute the onions for 2-3 minutes. Then stir in the carrots, celery, and garlic. Cook for another 3-5 minutes.
- Meanwhile, cut the beef into small 1/2-inch chunks. Push the veggies to the side of the pot and add the meat. Brown for 5 minutes, stirring once or twice. Then add in the broth, tomatoes, barley, herbs, crushed red pepper, and 1/2 teaspoon salt. Stir well.
- Cover the pot and bring to a boil. Lower the heat if needed and simmer until the barley is cooked and the beef is tender, stirring occasionally. About 30 minutes.
- Taste. Then season with salt and pepper as needed.

Nutrition

Calories: 373kcal, Carbohydrates: 27g, Protein: 30g, Fat: 16g, Saturated Fat: 6g, Cholesterol: 78mg, Sodium: 1563mg, Potassium: 903mg, Fiber: 6g, Sugar: 5g, Vitamin C: 7.7mg, Calcium: 103mg, Iron: 4.6mg

31.   The Perfect Greek Salad Dressing Recipe

Prep Time: 5 Minutes

Total Time: 5 Minutes

Servings: 12 Servings

Ingredients

- ¾ Cup Extra-Virgin Olive Oil
- 1 Large Juicy Lemon Zested And Juiced (About ¼ Cup)
- ¼ Cup Red Wine Vinegar
- 1 Teaspoon Dijon Mustard
- 1 Teaspoon Dried Oregano
- 1 Clove Garlic Minced
- ¼ Cup Crumbled Feta Optional
- Salt And Pepper

Instructions

- Set out a pint jar. Place the oil, lemon juice and zest, vinegar, Dijon mustard, oregano, and minced garlic in the jar.
- Cover and shake well to emulsify. Add the crumbled feta, if using, and shake again.
- Taste, then salt and pepper as needed. (I usually add about ½ teaspoon salt and ¼ teaspoon fresh cracked pepper.)

Nutrition

Calories: 132kcal, Carbohydrates: 1g, Protein: 1g, Fat: 14g, Saturatedfat: 2g, Cholesterol: 3mg, Sodium: 41mg, Potassium: 12mg, Fiber: 1g, Sugar: 1g, Vitamin A: 13iu, Vitamin C: 5mg, Calcium: 20mg, Iron: 1mg

32. Homemade Egg Drop Soup Recipe

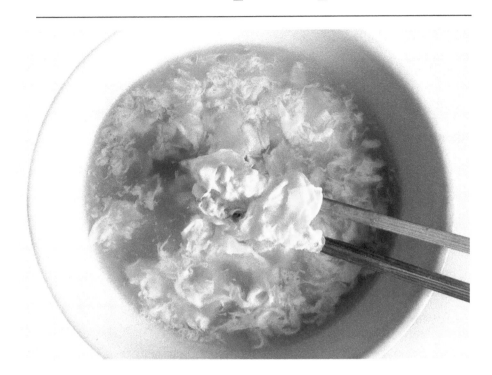

Prep Time: 5 Minutes

Cook Time: 10 Minutes

Total Time: 15 Minutes

Servings: 8

Ingredients

- 8 cups chicken broth
- 1/4 cup cornstarch (1/4 cup arrowroot powder for paleo)
- 1 1/2 tablespoon soy sauce (coconut aminos for paleo)
- 2 teaspoons sesame oil

- 1 teaspoon grated ginger
- 3/4 teaspoon garlic powder
- 1/4 teaspoon ground turmeric
- 6 large eggs

Instructions

- Add the chicken broth, cornstarch, soy sauce, sesame oil, grated ginger, garlic powder, and turmeric in a large saucepot. Whisk well. Then turn the heat on high and bring to a boil.
- In a small bowl, whisk the eggs well. Then stir the soup base to get it swirling and slowly pour the eggs into the soup. The eggs swirling into the soup will create ribbons of egg. Turn off the heat.
- Taste the soup and add salt and pepper to taste. Serve as-is, or garnish with chopped green onions and crunchy Chinese noodles.

Nutrition

Calories: 121kcal, Carbohydrates: 5.5g, Protein: 9.8g, Fat: 6.3g, Saturatedfat: 1.7g, Cholesterol: 140mg, Sodium: 985mg, Fiber: 0.1g, Sugar: 1.1g

33.   Crispy Brussel Sprouts Quinoa Salad Recipe

Prep Time: 15 Minutes

Cook Time: 30 Minutes

Total Time: 45 Minutes

Servings: 8

Ingredients

- 1 1/4 cup dried lentils, choose a more firm lentil type
- 2/3 cup dried quinoa
- 3 cups water
- 3/4 teaspoon curry powder
- 8 ounces Brussels sprouts
- 1 cup thinly sliced shallots, about 3-4
- 2 tablespoons olive oil
- 1/2 cup DeLallo Sun-Dried Peppers, chopped
- 1/2 cup scallions, chopped
- 1/2 lemon, juiced
- Salt and pepper

Instructions

- Preheat the oven to 400 degrees F. Place the quinoa and lentils in a medium stockpot with 3 cups of water, 1 teaspoon salt, and 3/4 teaspoon curry powder. Bring to a boil, then cover and reduce the heat to medium-low. Cook for 25-30 minutes until the quinoa is fluffy and the lentils are cooked, but firm. Remove from heat, but keep covered until ready to use.
- Meanwhile, cut the Brussels sprouts in half and slice thin. Place them on a rimmed baking sheet with the sliced shallots and drizzle with olive oil. Toss to coat then spread them out thin and salt and pepper. Bake for 20-25 minutes, until crispy.

- Fluff the quinoa and lentils and move to a large bowl. Add the crispy Brussels sprouts and shallots, chopped sweet peppers, chopped scallions, and the juice of half a lemon. Toss and salt and pepper to taste. Serve immediately.

Nutrition

Calories: 214kcal, Carbohydrates: 33g, Protein: 11g, Fat: 5g, Saturatedfat: 1g, Sodium: 18mg, Potassium: 546mg, Fiber: 12g, Sugar: 3g, Vitamin A: 900iu, Vitamin C: 30.9mg, Calcium: 44mg, Iron: 3.6mg

34. Harvest Salad (Cobb Style)

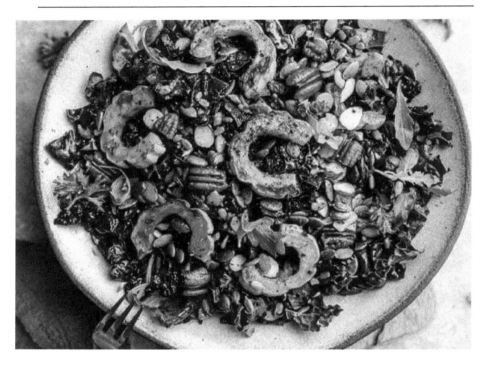

Prep Time: 20 Minutes

Cook Time: 2 Minutes

Total Time: 22 Minutes

Servings: 4

Ingredients

For The Cobb Salad:

- 2 romaine hearts roughly chopped
- 2 cups cooked chicken cut into cubes

- 2 cups roasted butternut squash cubes
- 6 slices thick-cut bacon cooked and crumbled
- 3 large hard-boiled eggs peeled and chopped
- 2 ripe avocadoes sliced
- 1 cup shelled pecans
- 1 tablespoon butter
- 1/4 teaspoon ground mustard
- 1/4 teaspoon garlic powder
- 1/4 teaspoon hot paprika
- 1/4 teaspoon salt

For The Creamy Corn And Poblano Dressing:

- 1 poblano pepper
- 1 clove garlic
- 2 ears corn on the cob cooked
- 2 limes juiced
- 1 teaspoon ground cumin
- 1 teaspoon salt
- 2/3 cup olive oil

Instructions

- Heat a skillet to medium-low heat. Melt the butter in the skillet, then add the pecans. Sprinkle the pecans with the ground mustard, garlic powder, paprika, and salt and toss to coat. Sauté for 3-5 minutes, stirring regularly to toast. Be careful not to burn the pecans.
- Pile the chopped romaine on a large platter. Arrange the chopped chicken, roasted butternut squash, bacon, pecans, eggs, and avocados in rows on top of the romaine.
- Preheat the oven to broil. Place the poblano pepper on a small baking sheet and set it on the top rack in the oven. Check the pepper every 1-2 minutes, turning when the skin is black and blistered. Remove the poblano from the oven when it's black on all sides. Place the pepper in a zip bag and allow it to steam for 10 minutes.
- Cut the corn off the cobs and place them in the blender. Add the garlic clove, lime juice, salt, and cumin. Once the pepper has steamed, removed the papery skin, stem, and seeds. Place the poblano flesh in the blender.

- Puree until smooth, then remove the ingredient cup from the lid and slowly pour in the olive oil to emulsify. Once the dressing is smooth and creamy, turn off the blender and pour the dressing into a serving bowl.

Nutrition

Calories: 860kcal, Carbohydrates: 20g, Protein: 16g, Fat: 83g, Saturatedfat: 17g, Cholesterol: 64mg, Sodium: 1139mg, Potassium: 741mg, Fiber: 6g, Sugar: 5g, Vitamin C: 52mg, Calcium: 94mg, Iron: 3mg

35. Greek Orzo Pasta Salad With Lemon Vinaigrette

Prep Time: 15 Minutes

Cook Time: 10 Minutes

Total Time: 25 Minutes

Servings: 8 Servings

Ingredients

- 1 pound dried orzo pasta
- 1 large red bell pepper seeded and diced
- 1 cup pitted olives (I used half kalamata and half green)
- 3 ounces sun-dried tomatoes chopped
- 1/3 cup diced red onion
- 1/3 cup chopped fresh basil
- 1/3 cup chopped fresh dill
- 1/3 cup chopped parsley
- For the Lemon Vinaigrette
- ½ cup fresh lemon juice
- ½ cup extra-virgin olive oil
- 1-2 teaspoons granulated sugar
- 1 clove garlic
- Salt and pepper

Instructions

- Set a large pot of salted water over high heat. Bring to a boil. Then cook the orzo as directed on the package. Drain.
- Meanwhile, set out a large salad bowl. Chop the bell pepper, onions, sun-dried tomatoes, and fresh herbs.
- In a small bowl (or measuring pitcher) whisk the lemon juice, olive oil, sugar, and garlic together. Set aside.

- Once the orzo is cooked and drained, place it in the salad bowl. Add in the bell peppers, olives, sun-dried tomatoes, onion, and all chopped herbs.
- Pour the lemon dressing over the salad and toss well. Cover and refrigerate until ready to serve.

Nutrition

Calories: 397kcal, Carbohydrates: 52g, Protein: 10g, Fat: 17g, Saturatedfat: 2g, Sodium: 296mg, Potassium: 583mg, Fiber: 4g, Sugar: 7g, Vitamin A: 1039iu, Vitamin C: 35mg, Calcium: 43mg, Iron: 2mg

36. Chunky Strawberry Salad With Poppyseed Dressing

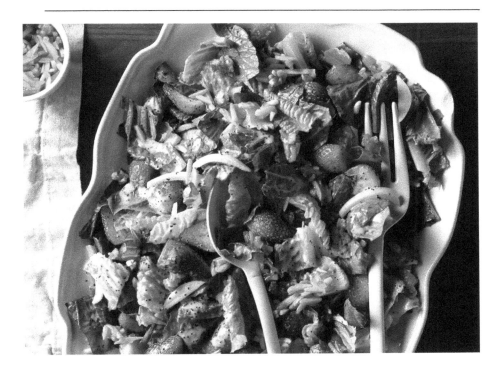

Prep Time: 15 Minutes

Cook Time: 0 Minutes

Total Time: 15 Minutes

Servings: 8 Servings

Ingredients

- 2 cups fresh strawberries hulled and sliced
- 6 ounces fresh baby spinach
- 1 cup sliced radishes
- ¾ cup chopped roasted macadamia nuts

- 1/3 cup crumbled chevre goat cheese
- ¼ sliced red onion
- ¼ cup store-bought poppyseed dressing (or homemade)

Instructions

- Slice the strawberries, radishes, and onion. Chop the macadamia nuts.
- Set out a large salad bowl. Add the spinach leaves, sliced strawberries, radishes, chopped nuts, and onions. Pour the dressing over the top and toss to coat.
- Then sprinkle the top with crumbled goat cheese, and gently toss again.

Nutrition

Calories: 166kcal, carbohydrates: 8g, protein: 4g, fat: 14g, saturatedfat: 3g, cholesterol: 6mg, sodium: 114mg, potassium: 259mg, fiber: 3g, sugar: 4g, vitamin a: 2091iu, vitamin c: 30mg, calcium: 54mg, iron: 1mg

37.   Wild Rice Salad With Blueberries And Herbs

Prep Time: 20 Minutes

Cook Time: 45 Minutes

Total Time: 1 Hour 5 Minutes

Servings: 12 Servings

Ingredients

- 2 cups dry wild rice
- 2 cups fresh blueberries
- 1 cup chopped scallions
- ½ cup shelled pistachios chopped
- ½ cup roughly chopped mint leaves
- ½ cup fresh chopped dill
- 1 large juicy orange zested and juiced
- 1 juicy lime zested and juiced
- ¼ cup olive oil
- 1 tablespoon honey or agave
- Salt and pepper

Instructions

- Cook the rice according to the package instructions. (For wild rice, usually, 2 cups of rice requires 6 cups of water and approximately 45-50 minutes of covered cook time.) Allow the rice to cool.

- Meanwhile, chop the herbs and pistachios. Then zest and juice the citrus.
- Move the cooled wild rice to a large salad bowl. Add the blueberries, scallions, chopped pistachios, mint, dill, orange zest, and lime zest.
- In a measuring pitcher, combine the orange juice, lime juice, olive oil, honey, 1 ¼ teaspoon salt, and ½ teaspoon ground black pepper. Whisk well then pour over the rice mixture. Toss to coat.
- Taste, then add additional salt and pepper if needed.
- Cover and refrigerate until ready to serve.

Nutrition

Calories: 126kcal, Carbohydrates: 15g, Protein: 3g, Fat: 7g, Saturated Fat: 1g, Sodium: 4mg, Potassium: 162mg, Fiber: 2g, Sugar: 6g, Vitamin A: 293iu, Vitamin C: 13mg, Calcium: 23mg, Iron: 1mg

38. Japanese Ginger Salad Dressing

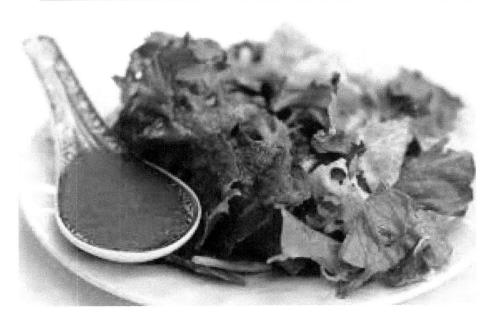

Prep Time: 10 Minutes

Total Time: 10 Minutes

Servings: 8 Servings

Ingredients

- 1 cup carrots roughly chopped
- ½ cup onion peeled and roughly chopped
- ¼ cup celery roughly chopped
- ½ cup rice vinegar
- 1/3 cup canola oil
- 3 tablespoons fresh grated ginger
- 2 tablespoons granulated sugar or honey

- 1-2 tablespoons soy sauce (I always buy GF and low sodium.)
- 1 small garlic clove

Instructions

- Roughly chop all the produce. Place in the blender.
- Add all other ingredients to the blender. If you are sensitive to sodium, start with 1 tablespoon of soy sauce. You can always add more if needed.
- Cover the blender and turn on high. Puree until smooth.
- Taste, then add more soy sauce if desired.
- Refrigerate until ready to serve.

Nutrition

Calories: 111kcal, Carbohydrates: 6g, Protein: 1g, Fat: 9g, Saturated Fat: 1g, Sodium: 140mg, Potassium: 90mg, Fiber: 1g, Sugar: 4g, Vitamin A: 2687iu, Vitamin C: 2mg, Calcium: 9mg, Iron: 1mg

39. Bubbly Taco Salad Bowls Recipe

Prep Time: 5 Minutes

Cook Time: 13 Minutes

Total Time: 18 Minutes

Servings: 4

Ingredients

- 4 10-12 inch flour tortillas (XL burrito size)
- 4 tablespoons vegetable oil (or any flavorless oil)

Instructions

- Preheat the oven to 350 degrees F. Set 4 oven-safe cereal bowls on a large rimmed baking sheet. Then set a large 12-14 inch skillet on the stovetop over medium heat.
- Pour 1 tablespoon oil into the skillet. Once hot, place the tortilla in the skillet. Use tongs to swirl the tortilla to coat it in oil, flip it over, and swirl it again. It needs to be coated in oil, on both sides, right away.
- Pan-fry the tortilla for 30-45 seconds per side, allowing it to puff up with large bubbles. (The bigger the bubbles the better!) Flip and repeat. Make sure the tortilla isn't turning dark. It should be golden-brown.
- Use tongs to move the tortilla to one of the cereal bowls. Tuck it down into the bottom of the bowl, to create a bowl shape with the tortilla. Take care not to deflate the bubbles.
- Repeat with the remaining three tortillas. Once all the tortillas are flash-fried and shaped into bowls, bake for 9-10 minutes until very crispy. Cool and fill.

Nutrition

Calories: 124kcal, Carbohydrates: 1g, Protein: 1g, Fat: 14g, Saturated Fat: 11g, Sodium: 7mg, Sugar: 1g

40. Hawaiian Macaroni Salad With Potatoes

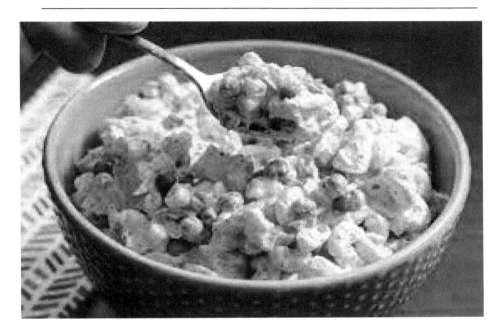

Prep Time: 15 Minutes

Cook Time: 14 Minutes

Total Time: 29 Minutes

Servings: 16

Ingredients

- 3 pounds Russet potatoes, peeled and chopped into 1-inch cubes
- 12 ounces dried macaroni noodles
- 1/2 cup shredded onion
- 1 large carrot, shredded
- 10 ounces frozen peas

- 1/2 cup chopped scallions
- 2 1/2 cups low fat mayonnaise
- 1 cup sweet pickle relish
- 1 tablespoon apple cider vinegar
- 1 teaspoon yellow mustard
- 1 teaspoon ground allspice
- Salt and pepper

Instructions

- Cut the potatoes into 1-inch cubes and place them in a large stockpot. Fill the pot with cold water until it is one inch over the top of the potatoes. Set the pot over high heat and bring to a boil. Once boiling, add 1 tablespoon salt. Then set the timer and cook the potatoes for 5 minutes. After 5 minutes, stir in the macaroni noodles and continue boiling for 6-8 minutes, until the pasta is al dente.
- Meanwhile, in a medium bowl mix the mayonnaise, sweet pickle relish including juices, apple cider vinegar, mustard, allspice, 1/2 teaspoon salt, and pepper to taste. Stir until smooth. Then use a grater to shred the onions and carrot.
- Drain the potatoes and macaroni in a colander and place in a large salad bowl. Add in the onion, carrots, peas, and scallions. Pour the dressing over the top and mix until well combined.
- Cover the potato macaroni salad and refrigerate for at least 4 hours. If you have time to make it ahead, it tastes even better on day two! Keep refrigerated in an airtight container for up to one week.

Nutrition

Calories: 268kcal, Carbohydrates: 43g, Protein: 5g, Fat: 8g, Saturatedfat: 1g, Cholesterol: 5mg, Sodium: 398mg, Potassium: 488mg, Fiber: 3g, Sugar: 8g, Vitamin A: 1015iu, Vitamin C: 13.3mg, Calcium: 28mg, Iron: 1.5mg

41.   The Ultimate Southern Chicken Salad Recipe

Prep Time: 20 Minutes

Cook Time: 3 Minutes

Total Time: 23 Minutes

Servings: 12 Servings

Ingredients

- 1 whole rotisserie chicken, about 5 cups chopped chicken
- 1 ¼ – 1 ½ cups mayonnaise
- 1 cup chopped celery
- 1 cup diced apple, a firm variety
- ½ cup sweet pickle relish
- ½ cup toasted almonds
- ½ cup chopped scallions
- 2 tablespoons dijon mustard
- 1 tablespoon fresh chopped dill
- Salt and pepper

Instructions

- Place the almonds in a small dry skillet. Set over medium heat. Toss and brown for 3-5 minutes, until golden. Turn off the heat. Meanwhile, chop all the produce.
- Remove the skin from the chicken and pull the cooked meat off the bones. Place all the chicken meat on a cutting board and roughly chop. Discard the skin and bones.
- Set out a large mixing bowl. Place the chicken in the bowl. Then add the mayonnaise, celery, diced apple, sweet pickle relish, toasted almonds, scallions, Dijon mustard, and dill.
- Stir well to evenly mix all the ingredients. Taste, then salt and pepper as needed.

- Cover and chill until ready to serve. (Chicken salad always tastes better after it has time to rest and chill. If possible, make a day ahead.)

Nutrition

Calories: 268kcal, Carbohydrates: 4g, Protein: 18g, Fat: 20g, Saturatedfat: 3g, Cholesterol: 59mg, Sodium: 274mg, Potassium: 154mg, Fiber: 1g, Sugar: 3g, Vitamin C: 1mg, Calcium: 11mg, Iron: 1mg

42. Ahi Poke Bowl Recipe

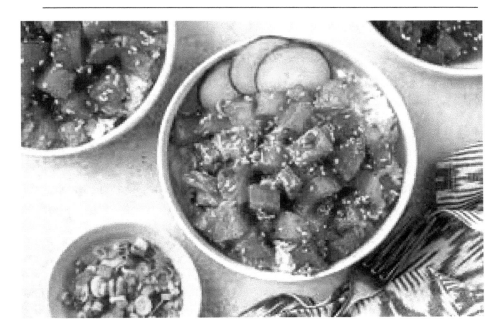

Prep Time: 15 Minutes

Cook Time: 20 Minutes

Total Time: 35 Minutes

Servings: 6 Servings

Ingredients

- 2 cups dried jasmine rice
- 1 pound sashimi-grade ahi tuna
- 3 tablespoons gluten-free soy sauce
- 2 teaspoons honey
- 1 teaspoon sesame oil
- 1/2 – 1 teaspoon wasabi paste
- 3/4 cup chopped green onions (green and white ends)
- 1 1/2 teaspoons sesame seeds

- 1 ripe avocado
- 1 bunch radishes
- 1 cup sprouts (alfalfa, broccoli, bean)
- Furikake Rice Seasoning

Instructions

- Pour the rice into a medium saucepot. Add 4 cups of water. Cover and bring to a boil. Once boiling, stir well. Then cover and lower the heat to medium-low. Simmer for 15-20 minutes until all the water is absorbed and there are air holes in the top of the rice. Remove from heat, fluff the rice with a fork, then cover to keep warm and set aside.
- Meanwhile, cut the ahi tuna steaks into 1/4 to 1/3 inch cubes. Place them in a bowl and add the soy sauce, honey, sesame, oil, and wasabi paste. Toss well to coat. Then stir in the chopped green onions and sesame seeds.
- Slice the avocado and radishes. Once the rice is cooked, assemble the bowls: Scoop a heaping portion of rice into 4-6 salad bowls. Spoon the ahi poke next to the rice and arrange sprouts and sliced radishes around the rice. Place several avocado slices over the top and sprinkle furikake on top.

Nutrition

Calories: 415kcal, Carbohydrates: 56g, Protein: 24g, Fat: 10g, Saturatedfat: 1g, Cholesterol: 28mg, Sodium: 543mg, Potassium: 496mg, Fiber: 3g, Sugar: 2g, Vitamin A: 1830iu, Vitamin C: 7.4mg, Calcium: 47mg, Iron: 2mg

43. Grandma's Best Ambrosia Salad Recipe

Prep Time: 15 Minutes

Cook Time: 0 Minutes

Total Time: 15 Minutes

Servings: 12

Ingredients

- 15 ounce can mandarin oranges
- 15 ounce can peach slices, drained
- 8 ounce can pineapple tidbits
- 5-ounce jar maraschino cherries stems removed
- ¾ cup fresh green grapes halved lengthwise
- ¾ cup sweetened coconut flakes
- ¾ cup mini marshmallows
- ½ cup chopped pecans, optional
- ¼ cup diced crystallized ginger, candied ginger
- 4 ounces sour cream
- 4 ounces cool whip
- Pinch of salt

Instructions

- Set a large colander in the sink. Pour the mandarin oranges, peaches, pineapple tidbits, and cherries into the colander.
- Once they are well-drained, chop each peach slice into 3-4 pieces. Remove all cherry stems, then cut the cherries in half.
- Cut the green grapes in half. Chop the pecans (if using) and dice the crystallized ginger pieces.
- Set out a large salad bowl. Pour the drained fruit into the bowl. Add the grapes, coconut, marshmallows, pecans, crystallized ginger, sour

cream, and cool whip. Add a good pinch of salt and gently mix the salad until everything is well incorporated.

- Cover and refrigerate until ready to serve. Can be made up to 7 days in advance.

Nutrition

Calories: 172kcal, Carbohydrates: 27g, Protein: 2g, Fat: 7g, Saturated Fat: 3g, Cholesterol: 6mg, Sodium: 35mg, Potassium: 218mg, Fiber: 3g, Sugar: 23g, Vitamin A: 675iu, Vitamin C: 16.5mg, Calcium: 40mg, Iron: 0.5mg

44. The Best Macaroni Salad Recipe

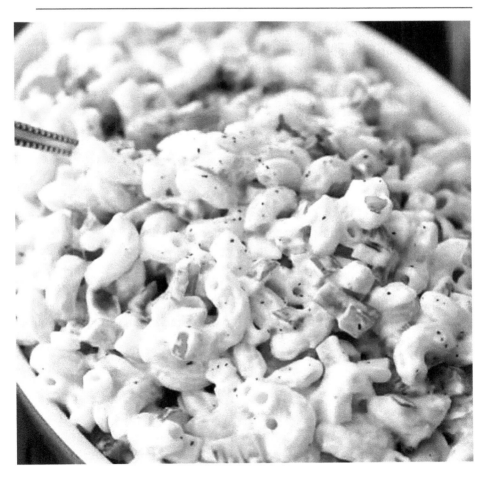

Prep Time: 15 Minutes

Cook Time: 10 Minutes

Total Time: 25 Minutes

Servings: 12 Servings

Ingredients

- 1 pound macaroni pasta
- 12 ounces roasted red pepper, (1 jar) drained and chopped
- 3/4 cup kale, finely chopped
- 1/2 cup cooked bacon, chopped
- 1/2 cup sweet pickle relish
- 1/2 cup scallions, chopped
- 1 1/2 cups mayonnaise, could be low fat
- 3 tablespoons apple cider vinegar
- 1 tablespoon granulated sugar
- 1 tablespoon hot sauce, i used frank's redhot
- 1 clove garlic, minced
- Salt and pepper

Instructions

- Bring a large pot of salted water to a boil. Cook the macaroni according to the package instructions, usually 7-10 minutes. Then drain and rinse with cold water.
- In a medium bowl mix the mayonnaise, apple cider vinegar, sugar, hot sauce, garlic, 1 teaspoon salt, and 1/2 teaspoon ground pepper.
- Pour the macaroni into a large bowl. Pour the dressing over the top. Then add the chopped roasted red peppers, kale, bacon, pickle relish, and scallions.
- Toss well to coat. Then refrigerate until ready to serve.

Nutrition

Calories: 362kcal, Carbohydrates: 34g, Protein: 5g, Fat: 22g, Saturated Fat: 3g, Cholesterol: 12mg, Sodium: 689mg, Potassium: 163mg, Fiber: 1g, Sugar: 5g, Vitamin A: 750iu, Vitamin C: 20mg, Calcium: 31mg, Iron: 1mg

45.   345. Fresh Peach Salad Recipe With Basil

Prep Time: 10 Minutes

Total Time: 10 Minutes

Servings: 6

Ingredients

- 4-6 ripe peaches pitted and cut into bite-size pieces
- 1 tablespoon honey
- 6 basil leaves thinly sliced
- 1/2 cup lemon chevre or plain chevre with a little lemon zest
- Pinch of salt

Instructions

- Place the peaches in a bowl. Drizzle with honey and sprinkle with salt. Toss to coat.
- Gently fold in basil and chevre. Serve immediately.

Nutrition

Calories: 99kcal, Carbohydrates: 12g, Protein: 4g, Fat: 4g, Saturatedfat: 2g, Cholesterol: 8mg, Sodium: 69mg, Potassium: 190mg, Fiber: 1g, Sugar: 11g, Vitamin A: 540iu, Vitamin C: 6.6mg, Calcium: 32mg, Iron: 0.6mg

46. Spicy Kani Salad Recipe

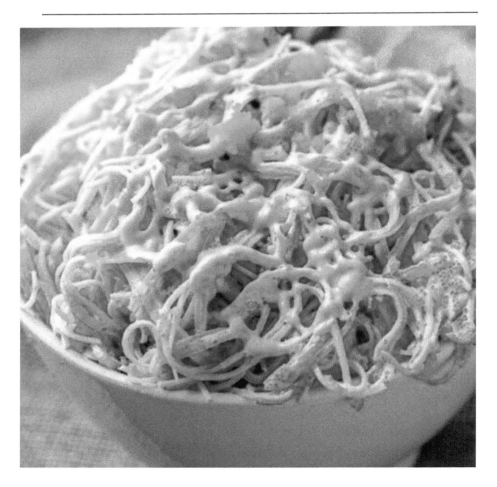

Prep Time: 30 Minutes

Cook Time: 0 Minutes

Total Time: 30 Minutes

Servings: 4

Ingredients

For The Dressing:

- 1/4 cup mayonnaise
- 2 tablespoon rice vinegar
- 1/2 teaspoon sugar
- 1 teaspoon sriracha sauce (chile sauce)
- 1/2 teaspoon paprika
- 1/2 teaspoon freshly grated ginger
- Pinch salt

For The Salad:

- 4 Kani sticks (1/2 pound imitation crab)
- 1 mango peeled and shredded
- 1 large cucumber (or three baby cucumbers) peeled and shredded
- 3/4 cup panko bread crumbs

Instructions

- Whisk the first seven ingredients together for the dressing. Taste for seasoning and salt and pepper as needed. Set aside.
- Shred the crab sticks by hand and place them in a large bowl. Shred the cucumber and mango in a food processor (or julienne by hand) and place in the bowl.
- Toss with the dressing and top with panko immediately before serving.

Nutrition

Calories: 178kcal, Carbohydrates: 16g, Protein: 2g, Fat: 11g, Saturated Fat: 1g, Cholesterol: 6mg, Sodium: 208mg, Potassium: 193mg, Fiber: 1g, Sugar: 8g, Vitamin A: 625iu, Vitamin C: 18.2mg, Calcium: 36mg, Iron: 0.8mg

47. Cucumber Salad

Prep Time: 15 Minutes

Cook Time: 0 Minutes

Total Time: 15 Minutes

Servings: 6

Ingredients

- 3 English cucumbers
- 1 tablespoon fresh chopped dill
- 1 clove garlic, minced
- 1 lemon, zested and juiced
- 1/2 cup plain greek yogurt
- 2 teaspoons granulated sugar
- Salt and pepper

Instructions

- Peel the cucumbers. Cut in half lengthwise. Then slice into thin pieces. Place the sliced cucumbers into a large bowl.
- Add the chopped dill, minced garlic, the zest of one lemon, 1 tablespoon of lemon juice, 1/2 cup plain greek yogurt, sugar, 1/2 teaspoon salt, and 1/4 teaspoon ground black pepper.
- Toss until the yogurt blends into a thin dressing. Taste, then salt and pepper as needed. Serve cold.

Nutrition

Calories: 38kcal, Carbohydrates: 7g, Protein: 2g, Fat: 0g, Saturatedfat: 0g, Cholesterol: 0mg, Sodium: 9mg, Potassium: 244mg, Fiber: 0g, Sugar: 4g, Vitamin A: 155iu, Vitamin C: 5.6mg, Calcium: 42mg, Iron: 0.4mg

48. Mexican Salad With Chipotle Shrimp

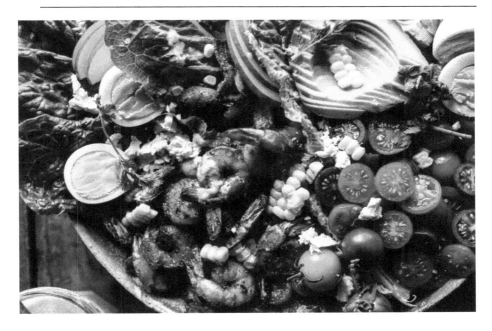

Prep Time: 15 Minutes

Cook Time: 10 Minutes

Total Time: 25 Minutes

Servings: 8

Ingredients

- 2-pound raw jumbo shrimp, peeled and cleaned (tail on or off)
- 8 cups chopped kale
- 4 ears corn on the cob, shucked
- 15 ounce can of black beans, drained
- 1-pint grape or cherry tomatoes halved
- 1 whole ripe avocado, peeled and chopped

97

- 2-3 whole chipotle peppers in adobo sauce
- 7 tablespoons fresh lime juice, divided
- 1/4 cup olive oil
- 1/4 cup mayonnaise
- 2 tablespoons honey
- 3 cloves garlic
- 1/2 teaspoon salt

Instructions

- Preheat the grill to medium heat. To a blender jar, add the chipotle peppers, 4 tablespoons of lime juice, olive oil, garlic, and salt. Cover and puree until smooth.
- Measure out 3 tablespoons of the chipotle puree and save it for the dressing. In a medium bowl, mix the shrimp and the remaining marinade, until well coated.
- In a separate small bowl, mix the 3 tablespoons of chipotle puree, 3 tablespoons lime juice, mayonnaise, and honey. Whisk until smooth. Then taste, and salt and pepper as needed.
- Prep all the veggies. Set out a large salad bowl. Add the kale. Then toss it with the dressing until well coated. (I like to massage the dressing into the kale by hand.) Then add in the black beans, tomatoes, and avocado.
- Place the shrimp and corn cobs on the grills. *If your shrimp are small they will fall through the grates. Either use a grill basket or place them on a piece of foil. Grill the shrimp for 3-5 minutes until pink. Grill the corn for 8-10 minutes rotating every 2 minutes.
- Once the corn is cool enough to handle, cut it off the cobs and add it to the salad. Then toss in the shrimp and serve.

Nutrition

Calories: 372kcal, Carbohydrates: 31g, Protein: 31g, Fat: 15g,Saturatedfat: 2g, Cholesterol: 288mg, Sodium: 1314mg, Potassium: 849mg, Fiber: 5g, Sugar: 9g, Vitamin C: 107.2mg, Calcium: 293mg, Iron: 5.1mg

49. Horiatiki (Greek Village Salad)

Prep Time: 10 Minutes

Cook Time: 0 Minutes

Total Time: 10 Minutes

Servings: 8

Ingredients

For The Greek Salad:

- 1 large English cucumber
- 1-pint grape tomatoes
- 1 bell pepper, any color
- 8-ounce feta cheese
- 1 cup pitted kalamata olives
- 1/2 cup fresh chopped mint leaves
- 1/4 cup sliced red onion
- For the Herb Vinaigrette:
- 4 tablespoons extra virgin olive oil
- 3 tablespoons red wine vinegar (or lemon juice)
- 1 clove garlic, minced
- 1 teaspoon dried oregano
- Salt and pepper

Instructions

- Set out a large salad bowl, and a small bowl for the vinaigrette. In the small bowl, whisk together the oil, vinegar, garlic, oregano, 1/2 teaspoon salt and 1/4 teaspoons ground black pepper. Set aside.
- Cut the cucumber into quarters, lengthwise. Then slice it into 1/2 inch chunks. Cut the grape tomatoes in half. Seed and chop the bell

pepper into 1/2 pieces. Cut the feta into 1/2 inch cubes. Chop the mint and slice the red onion.

- Place all the fresh produce in the large bowl. Pour the vinaigrette over the top. Gently toss to coat all the chunks in dressing. Then cover and refrigerate until ready to serve.

Nutrition

Calories: 186kcal, Carbohydrates: 6g, Protein: 5g, Fat: 15g, Saturatedfat: 5g, Cholesterol: 25mg, Sodium: 584mg, Potassium: 267mg, Fiber: 2g, Sugar: 4g, Vitamin C: 29.6mg, Calcium: 170mg, Iron: 0.9mg

50. Market Bean Salad Recipe

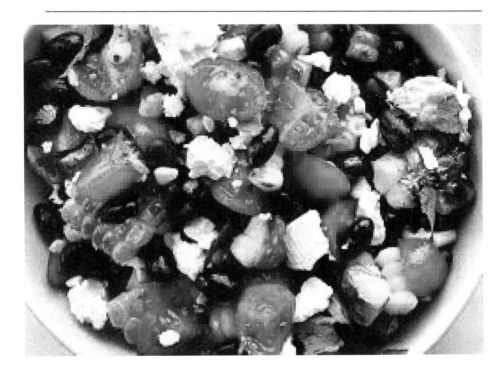

Prep Time: 15 Minutes

Cook Time: 40 Minutes

Total Time: 55 Minutes

Servings: 8

Ingredients

- 1 pound black-eyed peas, raw or frozen
- 1/2 pound white acre peas (field peas), raw or frozen
- 1/2 pound mixed sprouted peas and lentils
- 1-pint ripe cherry tomatoes
- 1/2 small red onion, chopped
- 2 cloves garlic, minced

- 1/3 cup flat-leaf parsley, chopped
- 2 tablespoons apple cider vinegar
- 1/4 cup extra virgin olive oil
- Salt and pepper

Instructions

- Place a large pot of water over high heat and bring to a boil. Salt the water liberally, then add the black-eyed peas. Simmer for 10 minutes, then add the white acre peas and simmer another 20-30 minutes, until both are soft and tender. Drain the peas in a colander and rinse under cold water to bring the temperature down. Shake to remove excess water.
- Place the cooked peas (beans) in a large mixing bowl. Add the sprouted peas, red onion, garlic, parsley, vinegar, and oil. Toss, then salt and pepper to taste and toss again.
- Cut the large cherry tomatoes in half and leave the small tomatoes whole. When ready to serve, pour the bean salad out on a serving platter then top with the cherry tomatoes.

Nutrition

Calories: 264kcal, Carbohydrates: 36g, Protein: 13g, Fat: 7g, Saturatedfat: 1g, Cholesterol: 0mg, Sodium: 14mg, Potassium: 650mg, Fiber: 14g, Sugar: 5g, Vitamin A: 735iu, Vitamin C: 30.4mg, Calcium: 49mg, Iron: 4.6mg

51. Steakhouse Salad

Prep Time: 10 Minutes

Total Time: 10 Minutes

Servings: 6

Ingredients

- 8 ounces romaine lettuce hearts
- 3 tablespoons Worcestershire sauce
- 3 tablespoons extra virgin olive oil
- 2 tablespoons fresh lemon juice
- 1 teaspoon minced garlic, fresh or from the jar
- 1/2 cup shaved Parmesan cheese
- Salt and pepper

Instructions

- Chop the romaine lettuce and place in a large salad bowl.
- Pour the Worcestershire sauce, olive oil, and lemon juice into a small jar. Add in the minced garlic, 1/2 teaspoon salt, and 1/4 teaspoon cracked black pepper. Whisk well.
- Pour the dressing over the lettuce and toss well to coat.
- Sprinkle the Parmesan cheese over the top and lightly toss. Serve immediately!

Nutrition

Calories: 109kcal, Carbohydrates: 3g, Protein: 3g, Fat: 9g, Saturatedfat: 2g, Cholesterol: 5mg, Sodium: 220mg, Potassium: 169mg, Fiber: 0g, Sugar: 1g, Vitamin A: 3355iu, Vitamin C: 4.7mg, Calcium: 120mg, Iron: 0.9mg

52. 3-Ingredient Almond Butter Balsamic Vinaigrette

Prep Time: 1 Minute

Total Time: 1 Minute

Servings: 4 Ounces

Ingredients

- 3 tablespoons almond butter
- 3 tablespoons balsamic vinegar
- 3 tablespoons water

Instructions

- Slowly whisk all ingredients until well blended. That's it. You're done!

Nutrition

Carbohydrates: 4g, Protein: 2g, Fat: 6g, Saturatedfat: 0g, Cholesterol: 0mg, Sodium: 4mg, Potassium: 103mg, Fiber: 1g, Sugar: 2g, Calcium: 45mg, Iron: 0.5mg

53. Chicken Gyro Salad With Creamy Tzatziki Sauce

Prep Time: 30 Minutes

Cook Time: 10 Minutes

Total Time: 40 Minutes

Servings: 4

Ingredients

For The Tzatziki Sauce:

- 1 cup plain Greek yogurt
- 1 hothouse cucumber
- 1 lemon, zested + 1 tablespoon juice
- 1 tablespoon olive oil
- 1 clove garlic, minced
- 1 tablespoon fresh chopped dill
- 1/2 teaspoon salt
- 1/4 teaspoon pepper
- For the Chicken:
- 1 pound boneless skinless chicken breast
- 1 tablespoon red wine vinegar
- 2 tablespoons olive oil
- 1 clove garlic, minced (large)
- 1 teaspoon dried oregano
- 1/2 teaspoon crushed dried rosemary
- Salt and pepper

For The Salad:

- 2 pieces flatbread
- 1 cup fresh mint leaves
- 1 small red onion, sliced thin

105

- 1 cup sliced cucumber
- 1 cup sliced tomato wedges
- 6 cups chopped romaine lettuce (2 cups for classic gyros)

Instructions

- Preheat the grill to high heat. Place the chicken in a baking dish and top with vinegar, oil, herbs, 1/2 teaspoon salt, and pepper to taste. Mix to coat and allow the chicken to marinate for at least 15 minutes.
- For the Tzatziki Sauce: Cut the cucumber in half. Use half for the tzatziki sauce and slice the remaining half for the salad. Peel half of the cucumber for the tzatziki sauce and grate it with a cheese grater. Wrap the shredded cucumber in a paper towel and squeeze it firmly over the sink to extract extra moisture. Then place the cumber in a bowl. Add the yogurt, zest on 1 lemon, 1 tablespoon lemon juice, olive oil, garlic, dill, salt, and pepper. Mix well and refrigerate until ready to serve.
- Once the grill is hot, lower the heat to medium and grill the chicken for approximately 5 minutes per side. Remove the chicken and allow it to rest 5 minutes before cutting.
- For the Salad: Pile chopped romaine in 4 bowls. Cut the flatbread into wedges. Slice the chicken and layer on top of each salad. Then arrange mint, red onion, cucumbers, tomato, flatbread wedges, and tzatziki sauce all around the chicken.

Nutrition

12ounces, Calories: 311kcal, Carbohydrates: 14g, Protein: 31g, Fat: 14g, Saturatedfat: 2g, Cholesterol: 75mg, Sodium: 458mg, Potassium: 1012mg, Fiber: 4g, Sugar: 6g, Vitamin C: 20.5mg, Calcium: 146mg, Iron: 2.3mg

54. Brazilian Chopped Salad

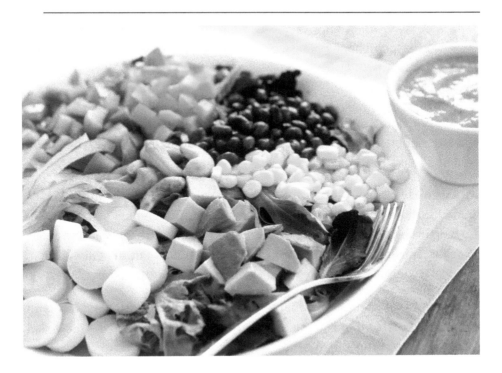

Prep Time: 15 Minutes

Total Time: 15 Minutes

Servings: 8

Ingredients

For The Brazilian Chopped Salad:

- 14 ounces hearts of palm
- 12 ounces cherry or grape tomatoes
- 1 fennel bulb
- 1 ripe avocado
- 1/2 small red onion
- 1/4 cup chopped mint

- For the Lime Vinaigrette:
- 1/4 cup fresh squeezed lime juice
- 1/4 cup olive oil
- 1 clove garlic, minced
- 1 teaspoon honey or agave
- Salt and pepper

Instructions

For The Vinaigrette: For the vinaigrette: Pour all the ingredients into a jar. Add 1 teaspoon salt and 1/2 teaspoon ground black pepper. Screw the lid on tight and shake to combine.

To Assemble: Drain The can of hearts of palm, then chop into 1/4-inch rounds. Cut the tomatoes in half. Cut the stems off the fennel bulb. Then cut the bulb in half and remove the core. Lay the fennel bulb halves flat, and slice into thin "shaved" pieces. Cut the avocado into chunks. Cut the onion half, in half again, then slice into thin strips. Finally, chop the fresh mint.

Place the shaved fennel on a large platter (or in a salad bowl.) Top with tomatoes, hearts of palm, onion, avocado, and mint. Drizzle the salad dressing over the top and toss.

Nutrition

1cup, calories: 182kcal, carbohydrates: 21g, protein: 2g, fat: 10g, saturatedfat: 1g, cholesterol: 0mg, sodium: 29mg, potassium: 1258mg, fiber: 3g, sugar: 10g, vitamin a: 375iu, vitamin c: 23mg, calcium: 36mg, iron: 1.6mg

55. Sun-Dried Tomato Chicken Pasta Salad

Prep Time: 15 Minutes

Cook Time: 8 Minutes

Total Time: 23 Minutes

Servings: 10

Ingredients

- 1 pound small dried pasta (any variety)
- 2 cups chopped leftover cooked chicken or rotisserie chicken
- 1 cup fresh baby spinach, packed
- 7 ounces sun-dried tomatoes in oil, drained
- 5 ounces pitted green olives, halved
- 1/3 cup chopped red onion
- 3/4 cup light mayonnaise
- 1/4 cup red wine vinegar
- 1 tablespoon dried Italian seasoning
- 1 clove garlic, peeled
- 1/4 teaspoon crushed red pepper

Instructions

- Place a large pot of salted water on the stovetop and bring to a boil. Cook the pasta according to package instructions. Drain the pasta in a colander and rinse with cold water to cool. Allow the paste to drain while you prep the remaining ingredients.
- Chop the sun-dried tomatoes into bite-sized pieces. Place the mayonnaise, red wine vinegar, Italian seasoning, garlic, crushed red pepper, and 1/4 cup chopped sun-dried tomatoes in the blender jar. Cover and puree.
- Place the cooled pasta, chopped chicken, spinach, remaining chopped sun-dried tomatoes, olives, and onions in a large salad bowl.

Add the creamy dressing and toss to coat. Cover the bowl with plastic wrap and refrigerate until ready to serve.

Nutrition

8ounces, Calories: 285kcal, Carbohydrates: 48g, Protein: 9g, Fat: 7g, Saturatedfat: 1g, Cholesterol: 2mg, Sodium: 401mg, Potassium: 823mg, Fiber: 4g, Sugar: 9g, Vitamin A: 545iu, Vitamin C: 9.1mg, Calcium: 52mg, Iron: 2.8mg

56. Tabouli With Feta And Endive

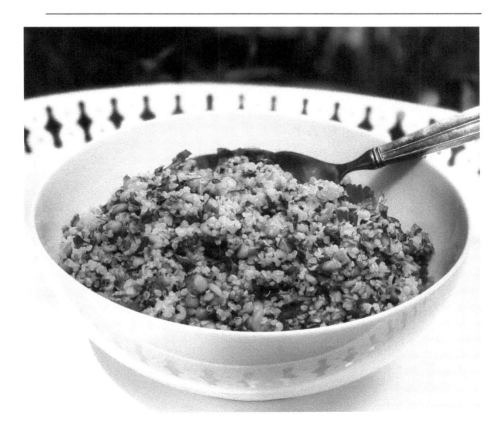

Prep Time: 20 Minutes

Cook Time: 5 Minutes

Total Time: 25mins

Servings: 12

Ingredients

- 1 cup bulgur wheat

- 1 1/2 cups boiling water
- 2 lemons, zested and juiced
- 1/3 cup extra virgin olive oil
- 1/4 teaspoon cayenne pepper
- 1 clove garlic (large), minced
- 2 1/2 teaspoon salt
- 1 bunch green onions, chopped (tops and bottoms)
- 1 bunch flat-leaf parsley, chopped
- 1 bunch mint leaves, chopped
- 1 English cucumber, chopped
- 2 pints cherry tomatoes, quartered (or 2 large tomatoes, diced)
- 1 cup crumbled feta cheese
- 8 heads endive (small)

Instructions

- In a large bowl, add the bulgur wheat, lemon zest and juice, oil, cayenne, garlic, and salt. Pour the boiling water over the top. Stir and allow it to sit for at least 1 hour.
- Wash the endive and cut off the bottoms. Carefully separate the leaves and set them aside.
- Chop all the herbs, cucumber, and tomatoes. Once the wheat has plumped up and absorbed the liquid, toss in the herbs, cumbers, and tomatoes. Then salt and pepper to taste.
- You can eat the tabouli immediately, but the flavor does develop if you give it a little time to sit. Scoop into endive leaves and sprinkle each with feta.

Nutrition

Calories: 202kcal, Carbohydrates: 25g, Protein: 8g, Fat: 9g, Saturatedfat: 2g, Cholesterol: 11mg, Sodium: 706mg, Potassium: 1260mg, Fiber: 12g, Sugar: 4g, Vitamin C: 54.7mg, Calcium: 248mg, Iron: 3.9mg

57. Raw Beet And Sweet Potato Salad

Prep Time: 10 Minutes

Total Time: 10 Minutes

Servings: 6

Ingredients

- 2 large sweet potatoes
- 1 bunch beets 3-4
- 4 scallions
- 1/2 cup toasted pepitas pumpkins seeds
- Garlic Lime Vinaigrette

Instructions

- Peel the sweet potatoes and beets. Then use a spiralizer to cut the veggies into long curly strips. Use a pair of kitchen shears to cut the pieces into manageable lengths.
- Mix the beet and sweet potato ribbons in a large bowl. Then cut the scallion tops on an angle to make long rings. Sprinkle the salad with scallions and pepitas. Serve with your favorite vinaigrette.

Nutrition

Calories: 169kcal, Carbohydrates: 11g, Protein: 2g, Fat: 13g, Saturatedfat: 2g, Cholesterol: 0mg, Sodium: 36mg, Potassium: 255mg, Fiber: 2g, Sugar: 3g, Vitamin A: 6225iu, Vitamin C: 3.2mg, Calcium: 23mg, Iron: 1mg

58. Healthy Rainbow Chopped Salad

Prep Time: 15 Minutes

Total Time: 15 Minutes

Servings: 4

Ingredients

For The Salad:

- 8-10 red radishes, chopped
- 1 orange bell pepper, seeded and chopped
- 1/2 pint yellow cherry tomatoes, quartered
- 2 small zucchini, chopped
- 1/4 small red cabbage, chopped
- 1 head romaine lettuce, chopped
- For the Avocado Chimichurri Vinaigrette:
- 1 soft avocado, peeled and pitted
- 1/2 cup chopped fresh parsley
- 1 tablespoon chopped fresh oregano
- 2-3 cloves garlic, minced
- 1/4 cup avocado oil or olive oil
- 2 tablespoons honey
- 2 tablespoons white wine vinegar
- 1/4 cup water, plus more as needed
- 1/2 teaspoon salt
- 1/4-1/2 teaspoon crushed red pepper

Instructions

- Place all the vinaigrette ingredients in a food processor or blender. Puree until smooth. Taste and salt as needed.
- Chop all vegetables and toss together in a large bowl. (Or you can lay them out in rainbow rows until just before serving.)

- Once ready to serve, pour the dressing over the salad and toss.

Nutrition

Calories: 321kcal, Carbohydrates: 30g, Protein: 6g, Fat: 22g, Saturatedfat: 2g, Cholesterol: 0mg, Sodium: 355mg, Potassium: 1304mg, Fiber: 10g, Sugar: 16g, Vitamin C: 113.7mg, Calcium: 137mg, Iron: 3.9mg

59. Thai Red Curry Grilled Chicken Salad

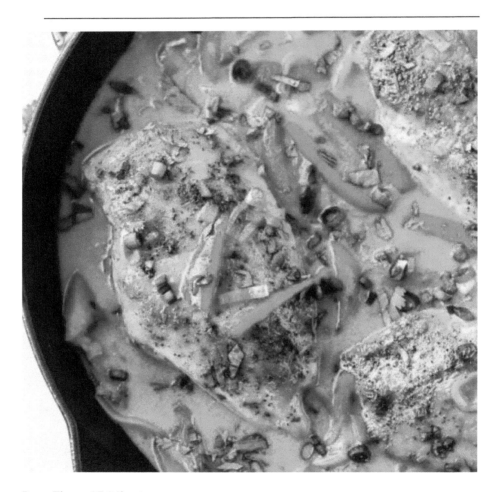

Prep Time: 15 Minutes

Cook Time: 10 Minutes

Total Time: 25 Minutes

Servings: 4

Ingredients

For The Thai Red Curry Grilled Chicken:

- 2 pounds boneless skinless chicken breast
- 4 ounces Panang Red Curry Paste
- For the Peanut Dressing:
- 1/3 cup creamy peanut butter
- 1/3 cup rice vinegar
- 1 tablespoon sesame oil
- 1 teaspoon honey
- 1 clove garlic
- For the Thai Red Curry Grilled Chicken Salad:
- 8 cups chopped napa cabbage (from one big cabbage)
- 1 mango, peeled and sliced thin
- 1 cup radishes, sliced
- 1 cup mini bell peppers, sliced
- 1/2 cup red onion, sliced
- 1/2 cup fresh cilantro leaves
- 1/4 cup roasted peanuts

Instructions

- Preheat the grill. Place the chicken in a baking dish. Rub the pieces of chicken on all sides with Panang red curry paste. Do not salt and pepper. Let the chicken marinate for at least 20 minutes.
- Place the ingredients for the dressing in a blender. Puree until smooth.
- Prep all the produce. Once the grill reaches 350-400 degrees F, grill the chicken for 5 minutes per side. Allow the chicken to rest another 5 minutes, before slicing into thin strips.
- Arrange the napa cabbage, mangos, and vegetables on salad plates. Top with sliced grilled chicken, cilantro, and peanuts. Serve each salad plate with a side of peanut dressing.

Nutrition

Calories: 575kcal, Carbohydrates: 24g, Protein: 59g, Fat: 27g,Saturatedfat: 5g, Cholesterol: 145mg, Sodium: 429mg, Potassium: 1602mg, Fiber: 6g, Sugar: 14g, Vitamin C: 76.6mg, Calcium: 203mg, Iron: 2.8mg

60.   Garlic Lime Roasted Shrimp Salad

Prep Time: 10 Minutes

Cook Time: 5 Minutes

Total Time: 15 Minutes

Servings: 10

Ingredients

- 2 pounds raw jumbo shrimp, peeled and deveined
- 2 tablespoons olive oil, divided
- 1 large English cucumber, chopped
- 1 firm avocado, peeled and chopped
- 1 lime, juiced
- 1 clove garlic, minced
- 1/4 cup fresh chopped mint leaves
- 2 tablespoons fresh chopped cilantro
- Salt and pepper

Instructions

- Preheat the oven to 450 degrees F. Line a large rimmed baking sheet with parchment paper. Pour the shrimp onto the baking sheet and drizzle with 1 tablespoon olive oil. Toss the shrimp in the oil and spread them out on the baking sheet. Sprinkle generously with salt and pepper.
- Roast the shrimp in the oven for 5-7 minutes, until pink. They should still be in the shape of C's. If they shrink to O's, you've overcooked them. Cool the shrimp on the baking sheet.

118

- Meanwhile, chop the cucumber and avocado in 3/4-inch chunks. Place the cucumber, avocado, minced garlic, chopped mint leaves, and cilantro in a salad bowl. Pour the lime juice and 1 tablespoon olive oil over the salad and toss well to coat. Taste, then salt and pepper as needed.
- Once the shrimp have cooled to room temperature, toss them into the salad. Cover and chill until ready to serve.

Nutrition

Calories: 155kcal, Carbohydrates: 3g, Protein: 19g, Fat: 7g, Saturatedfat: 1g, Cholesterol: 228mg, Sodium: 707mg, Potassium: 227mg, Fiber: 1g, Sugar: 0g, Vitamin A: 115iu, Vitamin C: 9mg, Calcium: 144mg, Iron: 2.2mg

Lightning Source UK Ltd.
Milton Keynes UK
UKHW020840040621
384920UK00001B/125